SORRY TO BOTHER YOU DOCTOR

ANDREW HAMILTON

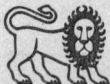

A LION PAPERBACK

Copyright © 1982 Andrew Hamilton

Published by
Lion Publishing plc
Icknield Way, Tring, Herts, England
ISBN 0 85648 332 X
Albatross Books
PO Box 320, Sutherland, NSW 2232, Australia
ISBN 0 86760 384 4

First edition 1982
Reprinted 1982, 1983, 1985

Author's Note
The stories in this book are mostly drawn from real
life; however, to preserved the anonymity of
those involved, not all details are accurate, and
the names of some people and places have been
altered.

Phototypeset by Input Typesetting Ltd, London
Printed and bound in Great Britain by
Collins, Glasgow

Contents

1
Wings of the morning

The lean figure in the bush-shirt, his arms waving, got smaller and smaller and was finally lost in the brightness of the brand new African day. How kind Geoff had been; bringing us those hundreds of miles in his pick-up, then wandering, quite unconcerned around the airport, carrying Barney's potty-chair in his hand, until the stewardess finally took pity on him and found a spare corner in the luggage-hold for it.

As we climbed into the azure sky, I felt the pattern of life was dropping away from us like the ground beneath. I drew back from the window. At first, Peter and Sarah could hardly keep still, but, after a time, both they and Elisabeth began to get drowsy, worn out with excitement and the days of travelling. I re-arranged Barney on my knee – at eighteen months he was already no lightweight – and leant back in my seat.

As if mingling with the subdued roar of the Viking's engines, I heard Ackroyd's voice again. 'You'll have to take her back to England, old man. That brucellosis, on top of the amoebic, has played havoc with her liver. If you don't, she could become a permanent invalid.'

'Well, he ought to know,' I'd thought, 'after all his years of tropical medicine.'

But it had been a hard blow. Elisabeth had been waiting outside, under the blue of a jacaranda.

'What did he say then?'

'He said we'd got to go to England.'

She'd looked at me and her eyes had been very soft. 'Andy dear, I'm so sorry.' Then, regaining her normal calm, 'Did you get all the order from Mac's? You remembered the porridge oats . . .?'

I thought, 'It's a miracle we're on this plane at all; well, perhaps not a miracle, that'd be pushing it, but, nevertheless, it's pretty amazing.'

We'd been almost broke, with not enough even for sea passages and the mission funds had been low as well. 'Sell the truck', the cable had said. What? Sell my precious hospital wagon, with its four-wheel drive and nice green coachwork? Just like that? Anyway, how was I to do it, stuck away in the mountains? Then the second wire had come, days late in the postboy's haversack. From Nairobi this time, sent by a settler friend: 'Bring truck Nairobi pronto firm offer white hunter.'

After the dusty trip down-country, I'd cleaned and polished that vehicle until it shone. The brawny hunter stalked round it.

'Give you £300,' he grunted. I nodded.

He whistled and a big Sikh came out with an oxy-acetylene torch and began cutting the body off. I might have saved myself such a lot of bother, I thought, only nobody's got around to telling me that white hunters only use open, canvas-covered trucks, to allow their bulky American clients to alight in comfort at the sight of game.

£300 was enough for sea passages but not for air fares, and I'd been longing to spare Elisabeth the heat of the Red Sea on board ship. So I tried the offices of all the air travel firms I knew in Nairobi to see if there might be any cheap fares going, but – no joy.

I was feeling at a low ebb when I came out of the last office and it was then I saw Harrison on the opposite side of Delamere Avenue. We'd met a few months before when he'd helped pick me as captain of East Africa against a South African touring rugby side, but I didn't feel I'd time to stop and talk just then. He spotted me, however, and came across.

'Hullo, Andy! What are you doing in Nairobi?'

'I'm afraid my wife is ill and I've been trying unsuccessfully to get some cheap air tickets home as we're short of cash.'

'My dear chap, I can fix that for you, come with me!'

On the way he explained that he was the civil air supervisor for Nairobi and sometimes people could get reduced rates with some companies, in cases of illness.

The manager at Airwork was brisk.

'Sure! Your wife's ill? How many are there of you?'

'Two adults, two children under eight and a baby.'

'Hmm – take you personnel rates – that'd come to £285. OK?'

'Yes, OK! And – thank you!'

The plane leaned over on a cushion of cloud as it banked to head north. I closed my eyes. Scenes like casually arranged shots of colour film began dancing through my head.

Eight years . . . it was eight years ago: we were on the cargo-boat out of Liverpool, U-boats were all around us, sinking ships in the convoy; now we were in New York, now the Panama Canal, through to the peaceful Pacific – Montevideo and the *Graf Spee* sticking out of the River Plate. Once again I heard that torpedo pass under us outside Walvis Bay . . . Now we had rounded the Cape, docked at Durban, got berths on a flying-boat up to Dar-es-Salaam, train to lake Victoria, paddle-boat . . . Now, at last we were in Kenya – we'd made it. Now I saw myself on safari, taking the bone out of the old man's smashed, infected hand . . . yes, it had been worthwhile coming to East Africa . . .

Whoops! The Viking must have hit an air-pocket. I opened my eyes and looked down through the window. Barney stirred and I dropped quietly back in the seat and closed my eyes again.

That patch of forest I'd just seen – wasn't that just like the bit where I'd gone on the leopard hunt, like an idiot, armed with an African bow (but with two hundred warriors), when our spotted friend had raided the sheep-hut at night? My mind wandered on . . .

I was seeing Geoff again, waving us off; what a superb surgeon he'd been in our primitive little hospital. I could see the neat job he'd made of that boy's head when he'd been brought in with his brain pulsating through the hole in his skull after he'd fallen out of a tree . . . Now we were in

Geoff's truck about to leave the hospital – there were the group of elders, a forest of hands reaching out to ours:

'*Saisere*! Goodbye Dokitare, goodbye Memsa'ab. If we do not meet again on earth we shall meet in heaven! Greet for us our brothers in England.' Then they were out of sight round the bend in the road . . .

Yes, 'brothers in England', what were things going to be like in England? My medical knowledge was dated; we were out of touch with the post-war way of life. It had been right to come to Africa and it was right to be going back, but where would we find a job so worth doing and within my capabilities?

One of the plane's engines sputtered, coughed and then resumed its even rhythm. It was enough to break the gloomy spell and a new refrain began to be intoned in my head – new, but with old familiar words:

'If I take the wings of the morning,
and dwell in the uttermost parts
  of the sea;
Even there shall thy hand lead me . . .'

I felt a deep sense of peace, the film show had faded from my mental screen and I drifted off into sleep . . .

The flight took three days, but that was nothing compared with the Red Sea and three weeks on a small passenger boat. We came down at Juba in the Sudan and there were huge cucumbers hanging from the thatched roof of the airstrip rest-house, then Khartoum, with the Nile flowing oilily past the hotel bedroom window, then Malta, Nice and finally Blackbushe in Hampshire, the terminal buildings looking like a collection of old army huts. Then, at last, there was my mother, standing in the doorway of the cottage, the smell of a good Scots high tea wafting through the hallway behind her.

That cottage in the Surrey hills was a complete bonus. Left, during the war, by Elisabeth's father – almost the only thing a poor country parson had to leave – and for all his family to share, it was unoccupied at just the right time for us. And, it had an Aga stove! O, Most Noble Aga! As the dank autumnal chill seeped into our African bones, there it stood, shining, immovable, day and night diffusing comforting warmth from the depths of its kindly, glowing heart. It cheered me when I returned, cold and rebuffed from a sally to the farmyard next-door.

'Hullo!' I'd said, brimming with tribal friendliness. 'We're just back in this country from Kenya . . .'

'Urr,' said the farm-hand and went to join his mate in the cowshed.

Now a tribesman would have spent a good five minutes asking after my personal health, that of my wife and children *and* our livestock, but I would do well to remember that this was Surrey, not the Rift Valley.

Two days later mother left us. That night Elisabeth and I sat on the kitchen chairs and reviewed our situation.

'I must get a job, love. I'd better look at the ads in the *British Medical Journal*. I'll do it in the morning.'

We said our prayers and reluctantly left the Aga for a cold bedroom.

I came down in the morning to make the tea. There was an envelope on the mat. I didn't know the handwriting. We sat in bed, and read the letter. The notepaper was headed 'Drs Charles Semple and Frederick Wilson' and the letter concluded by saying: '. . . so we are looking for a third partner. We heard that you had come back from abroad and wondered if you might be interested. Would you care to come down for an interview?'

The address was Wilverton-on-Sea.

'West Sussex, isn't it? How d'you fancy hob-nobbing with elderly schoolmistresses and retired colonels?' I asked Elisabeth.

It certainly wasn't what *I* had visualized, after our tribesfolk. When they were well, they were an athletic lot; in fact, one or two could even be in the Olympics in a year or two, I felt sure.

'I should go and see,' said Elisabeth. 'You know, it would be fine for the children . . .'

'And for you too, love,' I added.

So, we squandered several shillings on a long-distance phone-call and arranged an appointment with the doctors.

They insisted that they pay my train fare, which I thought was rather decent . . .

I got back late, dashed upstairs to say good night to the children and then came down to give Elisabeth my news.

'Surprisingly enough, they seemed to like me, and I must say I liked them too. They're working very hard and badly need help.'

'Yes, but what did they *say*?'

'Well,' I grinned all over my face, 'they've offered me the job! I told them I was a bit rusty and had wondered about a refresher course. Do you know what Semple said? "Can you write?" '

'Did you say you could?' said Elisabeth, pretending to look shocked.

'Oh, take it easy, it's not as bad as all that. Anyway they promised they wouldn't drop me in at the deep end. They said they'd show me the ins and outs of the Health Service and I could refer to them over any modern treatment I wasn't sure about, so there would be no risk to the patients.'

'Did they mention money?' Elisabeth asked quietly.

'I thought *I* was the one with Scottish forbears – yes, they did. Guess what they were prepared to pay me? £1,600 a year, for a trial period of six months, then, if we suited one another, they'd make me a junior partner!'

'£1,600? That would be three times our missionary allowance,' said Elisabeth. 'You'd have to be careful or you'd be paying income tax.'

'What, same as last time?' I queried, and we fell about laughing hysterically.

Perhaps the excitement of the occasion had something to do with it, but 'last time' had really been quite funny, that is, if income tax is ever funny. It was just before we left for Kenya that I got the tax demand. It was for £100. As our joint income only just topped £300, I reckoned they'd made a mistake. Anyway I wrote to the tax-man:

'Dear Sir,

'Since my wife's and my joint earnings for the past year only amount to £315, I feel that there must be some error and we surely could not be liable for tax. If you wish to pursue the matter, you will have to pursue us to Africa; we sail in three days' time.

'Yours faithfully . . .'

When we had recovered, Elisabeth asked, 'What did you say to them?'

'I said, "Naturally, I would like to talk it over with my wife".'

'Don't you feel you should have accepted, darling?' She looked at me a little anxiously.

'Well, I did find out that there is a tremendous shortage of openings in general practice, but we must be sure it's right. We felt we should look for a place with real needs, didn't we?'

'Don't the elderly have needs?' she asked, but I went on, 'They said they would wait for a few days and not offer the job to anyone else for the time being. But there's another small matter – what do we use for money, until we start? We need a house to live in, we'll need a car, we'll need medical equipment. And your clothes aren't quite what the professional man's wife is wearing these days!'

'The shorts you've got on at the moment wouldn't exactly impress the natives either!' she answered sweetly.

'Let's discuss it in the morning then, we're both tired,' I said finally.

It was quite early when I felt her stirring beside me. I'd been awake even earlier, thinking.

I whispered, 'Darling, do you remember what was almost the last thing old Geoff said to us? "Where God's finger points, his hand will open the way." Let's take the job.'

It was after that that things started moving. My dear old mum gave us some money, out of her bit of capital, to buy a car, though we'd never breathed a word to her about it. The local garage agreed to give us priority since I was a doctor; though, as their young salesman, who'd been evacuated to the States during the war, said, 'They're about as plentiful as hen's teeth'. Yet two weeks later it was delivered.

It turned out that the practice had all the medical gear I would want, and they even found us a furnished flat at a pretty nominal rent. Mind you, when I saw the flat, I realized why the rent was nominal – but it suited our pocket. As for clothes – well, the natives would just have to take us as they found us.

A week later, with our scanty possessions packed up and sent by rail, we piled into our brand new little Hillman Minx and prepared to set off. As we paused at the gate, I smiled over at Elisabeth, 'Wilverton, here we come!'

2
What makes them tick

'There's an urgent call for you, Dr Hamilton.'

I looked up at the kindly grey eyes. 'Right-ho. Just a moment and I'll be on my way.'

You didn't question Miss Spencer – at least, I didn't. She'd been with the practice, 'man and boy', for forty years, right from the day of the pony-trap. I hadn't been with it for forty days.

I put the top back on my fountain-pen, the medical history card back in its envelope and picked up my bag. Miss Spencer handed me a slip of paper, 'Albert Judd, 3 Camberley Gardens'.

'I've put directions on the back, how to get there,' she said. She knew I didn't yet know my way about too well.

I walked smartly out to the car park. As I got in I smelt the newness of the Minx.

'Lucky having a new car,' I thought. 'It's the first new one I've ever had.'

With the help of Miss Spencer's map I was able to do the three-quarters of a mile to Camberley Gardens, through narrow streets, in about four minutes. I ran up the steps of No. 3, banged the knocker and walked in. A face looked over the upstairs balustrade; it was an anxious face, framed in grey hair.

'I'm Dr Hamilton,' I called up.

'Oh doctor, I am glad you've come. Mr Judd didn't come down for his breakfast, so I went up and knocked on his door, but he wouldn't answer and I can't get the door open.'

I pushed the door, it opened about an inch and then wouldn't budge. I listened and could hear stertorous breathing inside.

'Look,' I said to the landlady, 'will you ring 999 for the ambulance, while I try to get into his room?'

I dropped my bag at the bedroom door, ran down the stairs and out into the front garden. I was right: there was a one-storey annexe at the side, with a flat roof beneath what I guessed was Mr Judd's window. I pulled myself up the drain-pipe and over a little parapet, then trod gingerly on a tarred roof to the window. I wiped away the salt encrusting it and peered through. I could just make out the form of Mr Judd, full length on the floor, his head pressed hard up against the door.

The bottom half of the window wouldn't budge, but I managed to lever open the top and force it down a foot. I wriggled through and dived on to my hands on the dressing-table, scattering an assortment of studs, cuff-links, brushes and combs over the floor.

Mr Judd's mouth was in a pool of vomit. His neck and face were a deep purple. I hauled him back from the door, which was no mean feat as he must have weighed a good sixteen stones, and turned his head gently to one side. His breathing improved and the blue colour changed gradually to pink.

I opened the door, got my bag and listened to his heart with my stethoscope. The beat was surprisingly strong and regular. I was just gently moving his arms and legs, when I heard a cheery voice through the door.

'Hullo, doc. What've we got then?'

In came two men dressed in blue uniforms, brisk, efficient and reassuring.

'Stroke,' I said, 'but I think he may make it. His general condition doesn't seem too bad.'

Those slimly-built ambulance men moved the massive inert figure on to a stretcher.

'Can I give you a hand?'

'No thanks, doc,' and unsaid, I imagine, 'You'd only be a right nuisance anyway!'

They carried him down the stairs in an effortless manner. I stood at the door until the sound of the ambulance bell died away, then turned back into the house to say a word of comfort to the landlady, before walking out into the winter sunshine. I was feeling warmed and comforted. I might be a bit of a back-number medically but I still had my uses.

I felt much less warmed and comforted when I heaved my six-foot bulk out of the Minx at my next call and discovered an eight-inch split in the back of Uncle Willie's trousers.

A cousin of mine in Scotland had heard of our return and, guessing that we might not be equipped for the rigours of the English climate, had sent me one of her father's suits (smelling strongly of mothballs). Sadly, he had died while we were abroad, but, canny Scot that she was, my cousin had put by the best of his clothes, in case someone was in need.

Someone *was* – but Uncle Willie has been five feet four and 'weel' covered. The trousers were forty-four inches round the waist but had only a twenty-eight-inch leg. Dr Semple told me of a good little tailor who performed wonders on that suit. Unfortunately, he took the seat of the trousers in a *wee* bit too much. I had to make an emergency stop for repairs at the flat before resuming my round.

Visiting went on till late afternoon and there was just time to nip in again for a cup of tea to revive me for evening surgery. Elisabeth had a tray ready in the bay-window. Barney was busy wrecking and rebuilding houses of wooden bricks on the floor. She turned her face to me, away from the window, as I came into the room.

'It's amazing how many poor, decrepit, old folk there are here.'

I looked out. An empty bath-chair was being trundled by. I recognized the charioteer. Bates was a patient of ours. I'd

16

met him once in the surgery when he'd been collecting a prescription for one of his clients.

He was an ex-Guardsman of six feet four and about seventeen stones, with a face like a genial gargoyle. Bath-chairs were mere toys in his massive hands. Gradients meant nothing to him; uphill or down, his passengers enjoyed an even military pace. They positively queued for his services. You would never have described him as a talkative man and this was probably just as well.

Even in ordinary conversation, his stentorian, parade-ground voice had a deep baying resonance which would have had an occupant of his chair nervously reaching for her hearing-aid to adjust the volume, had he indulged in conversation. He passed our way quite frequently, but the only time I heard him give tongue was in descriptive barrack-room phrases when he slipped on a dog's visiting card and projected bath-chair and occupant into a laurel bush.

The local geography must have had a good deal to do with the longevity of the residents of Wilverton. The town was built on seven hills like Rome, but that is where any resemblance ceased, unless Rome also has an unpredictable bus service and an equable climate. Healthy exertion in the open air thus became inevitable, to the benefit of the population.

People came to Wilverton to die and then forgot why they came. From all directions they would walk to our central surgery, nicely situated where four roads met. Thirty per cent of the patients were over retirement age, and eighty year-olds two-a-penny.

Everyone knew the surgery as St Arkel, though who he was no one could ever tell me. The building was a rather charming, old, converted stables which had belonged to a big house up a drive among some trees. My consulting room had been the tack-room. Pegs and hooks still stood out of walls and ceiling. Sarcastic patients sometimes asked if we used them for orthopaedic manipulations.

I greeted our secretary as I went in.

'Evening, Miss Spencer.'

'Good evening, doctor. Your records are on your desk.'

I looked at the pile. The first one had the name 'Mrs Evelyn Farley'. My heart sank.

We got on all right, Mrs Farley and I, but I was finding a visit a week becoming a strain. She had attached herself quite firmly to me. I think she needed a fresh audience. Reluctantly I pressed the buzzer.

'Good evening, Mrs Farley, do sit down.' Her chair creaked in protest. 'Well now, what's the trouble?'

'Doctor, it's the knees.'

It was understandable; arthritis and years of carrying that weight were telling at last.

Attempts at persuading Mrs Farley to diet never really got off the ground – she ate her diet and then had a 'real' meal after. 'Knees' however were really only the opening gambit; barely drawing breath she carried on.

'And I get this terrible wind after meals, doctor, up *and* down; I lose my puff on these hills, and there's this awful buzzing in my ears. Would you be good enough to have a look at them?'

If I hadn't already been acquainted with this cataract of symptoms I would have been overwhelmed by now. I examined her knees, her heart and her ears, then hastily began to write out a prescription, but I was too late.

'I've never been the same since my operation. I was on the table three hours and then I got the death rattles.'

I shuddered as she gave me a demonstration. Her notes indicated that this experience had occurred twenty-five years ago so I tried a quick counter.

'I don't think that could be affecting you now, Mrs Farley. I will give you something to help your knees.'

But I was losing ground. Mrs Farley was on her feet and heading for the examination-room. 'I think you should look at the scar, doctor, it doesn't feel right.'

I groaned quietly as she closed the door, visualizing the time-lag while she removed layer after layer of clothing. I managed to see two more patients before a discreet cough within called me back to harsh realities.

There was an advantage in a separate dressing-room. Un-dressing and dressing time could be put to good use. I'd heard that there were dangers though. Dr Semple had sent a quiet little man along the short corridor to his examination-room with instructions to undress and get up on the couch. It was nearly his last case of the morning.

At noon, the secretary was clearing Dr Semple's desk before going home to have lunch. She heard a quiet uncomplaining voice coming from the room: 'I feel better now, may I get down?'

I rang for Miss Spencer to chaperone me, took a deep breath and went into the little room.

'No doctor, not there, *there*. That's where the pain is.'

I wasn't surprised. Mrs Farley zealously imbibed large amounts of her own brand of laxative, calculated to give a camel colic.

'I don't think there is anything wrong with the scar, Mrs Farley. I advise you not to take medicine unless ordered by us. It could upset you. I'll write that prescription for you.'

When she came out at last I handed her a folded paper.

'Now take this and it will help your knees. Please try to eat less; if you are lighter, your knees won't have to carry so much.'

'Thank you, doctor.' Mrs Farley was almost through the door when she turned.

'You know we don't like bothering you doctors, but you *are* a necessary evil.' I smiled – she meant it kindly.

An hour later, I pressed the buzzer yet once more. The telephone rang.

'That's your lot, doctor,' said Miss Spencer.

I wrote some referrals, picked up my stethoscope, auriscope and ophthalmoscope, put them in my bag and went out to the waiting-room. Mrs Farley was still there.

'Hullo, not gone yet?'

'No, doctor. I'm waiting for Tommy to see me home.'

At that moment a bright-faced boy came in from the street.

'Come for your gran, then?'

'It's my *mum* not my gran, doctor,' he answered swiftly. 'Hullo Mum, sorry I'm late. Twinkle was naughty. I couldn't groom him, he wouldn't stand still.'

I noticed for the first time his grubby jodhpurs and the battered riding-hat he had in his hand.

'Now then you two – you don't live far from me, want to have a lift home?'

'Thanks, doc,' he answered quickly before his mother interposed, 'We shouldn't bother you, doctor.'

'That's all right.'

I knew they didn't live all that near me but three minutes' ride in a car was twenty-five on foot for Mrs Farley with her groggy knees. On the way home Tommy told me he was mad on ponies. Mum couldn't afford it, especially since Dad died, so he helped muck out at the local riding school and got rides as a reward.

We got to Castleton Row, a down-at-heel Victorian terrace some rows behind the front, stuccoed and four-storied, where formerly servants inhabited the basements and attics and gentry occupied the rest. We stopped at number twelve.

'Come in for a cup of tea, doctor?' Mrs Farley pleaded.

Home and supper were very desirable, but I didn't want to disappoint her.

'Thank you very much. Lead the way then, Tommy.'

He rushed down the basement steps. I heard him shout.

'Sis, make the tea, Dr Hamilton's coming with Mum.'

A quiet-looking girl of about eighteen met us in the passage.

'Good evening doctor, please come in to the front room while I bring some tea.'

I looked around. Everything was very neat and tidy though shabby. The floral linen covers on the three-piece suite were quite bright but then not much sunlight got in to fade them. 'Sis' brought in a tea-tray. I guessed that this was the best china. My mind went back to Kenya when we entertained a lady reporter from the *East Africa Standard* on our mission station. We had regaled her on our last tin of salmon and used our best wedding tea-set. Afterwards she wrote a report on her visit headed 'Missionaries live well'.

While I sipped my hot tea, Julia and Tommy told me quite naturally about themselves. I began to feel the strong bond that existed in this family.

'You see doctor, Mum brought us up by herself when Dad died. She used to clean at the Merivale Hotel until her knees got too bad. Then she went on the assistance. I do a job in a nursing home now, but I'm going to hospital to do proper training this year,' she finished proudly.

Mum looked just as proud. I felt ashamed. This was another Mrs Farley – not the one I thought I knew. She must be a careful mother who had kept her family together. Perhaps she found it a relief unloading her troubles on us. So what? We could take it.

As Julia spoke, my eyes wandered round the room. I saw a red leather Bible on a side-table. Mrs Farley followed my eyes.

'That's what helps us, doctor. We all read together each morning with Scripture notes. It makes all the difference.'

'So it does for me, Mrs Farley. Well, I'd better push off now. My wife will wonder where I am. Thanks for the tea.'

'Goodbye, doctor,' said Julia and Tommy together.

Elisabeth met me at the flat door.

'Andy, where have you been? The surgery rang for you but I had to say you weren't back yet.'

'I've been doing some research.'

'Research? What sort of research, for goodness' sake?'

'Oh, just into what makes patients tick.'

'Well, there's one who isn't ticking too well at the moment,' said Elisabeth. 'There's a call for a Mr Vanborough. He can't get his breath. Miss Spencer says he has a bad heart and would you go as soon as you come in. I'm sorry, I had smoked haddock ready for your tea.'

Smoked haddock had been my favourite delicacy since boyhood. As I came home from school in London, I would stand in the rush-hour trains ruminating on it, and the mental aroma would make me oblivious to stinking pipes and damp coats. I sighed.

'Oh well, keep it warm for me. Won't be long – I hope.'

I drove away through the lamp-lit streets to the north end of the town. I already knew Mr Vanborough. If he was breathless, it meant he was in acute heart failure and needed help urgently.

'He's that bad, doctor,' Mrs Vanborough anxiously led me along the passage. 'He simply can't breathe.'

Mr Vanborough was sitting on the edge of the bed, blue and wheezing. A trickle of fluid dropped from his mouth as he coughed. I sucked up an ampoule of morphia into a syringe, swabbed his arm and stuck in the needle. He got the full quarter grain.

I sat down with him on the edge of the bed and held his wrist. Ostensibly I was taking his pulse, but I was really trying to still the panic in him by a little human contact. His heart was flagging, fear was an enemy. Part of the work of the morphia was to relieve that fear, I was adding my help as well.

In a quarter of an hour something wonderful was happening. His breathing had eased and he had stopped coughing. A few moments more and his colour was better and he looked up, smiled and said quietly, 'Not too bad now, doctor.'

While I had been sitting there, I had had the distinct feeling of eyes watching me. Now I had time to look over the end of the bed. A large heron stood there staring at me with sardonic eyes which didn't wink. He was stuffed and in a glass case. I turned my head. On the mantelshelf a pair of owls looked down disapprovingly.

I felt Mr Vanborough's wrist. His pulse, instead of being thready and irregular, was now stronger, steady and slow. The action of morphia alone never ceased to amaze me. There are lots more drugs now. Diuretics to relieve the fluid congesting the lungs. Aminophyllin to expand the passages. But still nothing surpasses morphia for the treatment of acute congestive heart failure.

I stood up.

'You'll be all right now – I'll come and see you in the morning. Mind you sit well up in bed and don't slide down, it will help your heart.'

Mr Vanborough was quite alert, in spite of the morphia. He noticed me as I looked reprovingly at the heron with its supercilious look. He became quite talkative.

'Wouldn't be allowed to take 'em now, doctor. Had him and the owls since I was a boy. Shot the heron on the marshes. Shouldn't have done, but we never thought about it in those days. They were stuffed by Mr Bristow. We lived in East Sussex then. Have you heard of him?'

I had. He'd been a taxidermist suspected of importing rare bird skins and stuffing them and then claiming he'd caught them himself in Sussex. They became known as the 'Hastings Rarities'. I knew a doctor in that part of the world who had Bristow's daughters as patients and he'd once told me how grieved they were at the besmirching of their father's name after his death.

'You know, doctor,' went on Mr Vanborough quietly, 'Mr Bristow never tried to take in those ornithologists. He wouldn't have. I knew him. Honest and a good man he was. He caught those birds. There was a lot of unusually stormy weather and winds off the continent in those days. I reckon they were blown across the Channel. He caught 'em all right and he stuffed them, beautifully.'

I could have been interested but my stomach was empty and my thoughts now more of smoked haddock than birds.

'Well, see you in the morning, Mr Vanborough.'

Next day, he was sitting up in a chair, quite recovered. As I packed up my stethoscope and blood pressure apparatus, he put a hand on my arm.

'Doctor, I could see you were interested in the heron and the owls. You were, weren't you? Well, I'm an old man and they just collect dust for the missus. Would you do me a favour and take 'em away, if you like 'em?'

I gasped. It was a tempting offer. Peter, although he was not quite eight, was already becoming quite a naturalist and he'd be over the moon with a stuffed heron and two owls to start a collection. I didn't even think about our congested flat, the big glass case and what Elisabeth's comment would be.

'Thank you very much, Mr Vanborough. Are you sure?'

'You take 'em, doctor – I'd be pleased to think you'd appreciate 'em.'

I carried them out carefully and stowed them on the back seat of the Minx.

I'd had spears and honey and even a goat as presents in the past – but never before had I been given *a stuffed heron*.

3
'For everything there is a season'

'You'll see a bit of everything here, in spite of any first impressions you may have got. Ecclesiastes chapter three verse two would just about cover it.' Fred smiled comfortingly.

My knowledge of the Old Testament didn't compare with his so I just said, 'I believe you.'

We were having dinner with my partner Fred Wilson and his wife Grace. It was only a few months since I'd accepted his invitation to join the practice, after my eight years at the mission hospital in Kenya. I was finding the transition a bit drastic. Fred was doing his best to ease off some of my irksome reactions to work at Wilverton.

As we talked about it I realized – there wasn't much to grumble about. People are just people the world over and if he cares about them, a doctor soon builds up a satisfying relationship wherever he is. Perhaps it took a little longer in Africa because of the time needed to understand one another's culture. The folks in this Sussex town were already making us feel at home – that we belonged. That was it – 'belonging'. You could belong here – it wasn't too impersonal.

Wilverton was a compact little town of about 30,000 inhabitants. The older buildings near the front were a mixture of Georgian and Victorian periods, mostly houses and hotels now, with rather decayed terraces behind. Further back there were houses built just after the First World War and the larger shopping centre of the town lay there, where our surgery was placed. The council estate stood on the north side with the flats. Our hospital looked down from the east and below it on the coastline was the small harbour where fishing boats moored and the sailing club had its headquarters, handy for the hospital when half-drowned members of the club needed resuscitation!

In the lanes around the foot of the Downs were farmhouses and hamlets built of knapped flints where the most outlying of our patients lived. The road to London and the railway skirted the western end of the Downs while the other main road headed east up a valley and on over the Downs towards Brighton.

At four o'clock next morning I picked up the phone and heard a girl's frightened voice.

'Can you come and see my sister, doctor? She's got an awful pain in her stomach.'

'What is her name and her address please?'

'Mrs Judy Spinks, 25 Grimble Court.'

'All right, I'll be with you as soon as I can.'

'Thank you, doctor.'

With that she put the phone down. There was just no chance to get any further information.

As I drove through the dark streets, the sky began to brighten to the east behind the Downs, and the light just caught the top of the block of flats for which I was heading. As I went into the bedroom I wished most fervently she had told me more – at least one vital fact.

The young woman on the bed was obviously well on in labour and I hadn't got my midder bag. In fact I hadn't even got my ordinary emergency bag – it was down below in the car. I wasn't at my brightest at 4 a.m., and I'd been expecting a case of acute gastritis or possibly an appendix. There was no time, I felt, even to get my emergency bag.

I washed and did an internal examination. She was fully dilated and the head was well down. Thank goodness, it was a normal presentation and the foetal heart was steady. At that moment Judy Spinks had a contraction and she let out a little cry through her clenched teeth.

I turned to her sister.

'Is there anyone else who could give me a hand?'

'Mum lives up on the next floor.'

'Well, you get her down at once. Tell her your sister's just about to have her baby.'

She stared at me wide-eyed and then turned and ran out of the flat.

For a moment a feeling of desperation – almost panic – took hold of me. I'd become dependent in a comparatively short space of time on the ministrations of a midwife, on sterile equipment, an anaesthetic and all the paraphernalia of a nice, orderly, aseptic delivery. Then my mind flashed back to a room in a small brick building, lit by the flickering light of a hurricane lamp, and a fight to save a baby with the help of forceps and chloroform, administered by a half-trained African nurse. We won, but it was a near thing, with a mother who'd been on the trail for twenty-four hours, in obstructed labour.

I looked down at this young woman, so near to giving birth, doing her part instinctively and trusting me to do mine.

'Come on Hamilton, get on with it!' I said to myself.

Mum arrived, confused and bleary-eyed.

'Your daughter's baby is nearly here,' I snapped.

'It wasn't due for a fortnight,' she protested.

'Will you go out to the kitchen, find a pair of scissors and reel of thread, and boil them up in a pan for me?'

She went off dumbly.

I sent the sister down to phone for the midwife and I ransacked the linen cupboard, before going back to the bedside.

The head was appearing. Judy's Mum returned.

'Can't find any scissors.'

'Well, boil up a kitchen knife,' I said quickly.

Judy did all she was told except that she pushed too hard at the end and the baby came with a rush. I tied the cord and sawed it through with the knife. The placenta followed and her uterus tightened up beautifully. I wrapped the baby in a towel and showed Judy.

'Coo, Bert'll be pleased! 'E's on nights at the fire station.

Wasn't expecting the baby for two weeks. We 'aven't even got a cot yet.'

Mum had collapsed in a chair. I held out the baby to her. 'Take a look at your grandson.'

Her eyes filled. 'My, my', was all she could manage, smiling through her tears. I had just cleared everything up when the midwife arrived.

'How are we doing then?' she asked briskly.

'All shipshape – even without benefit of midwife,' I said, rather cockily.

I left her to take over and departed.

Breakfast revived me and I went off as usual to surgery.

At three o'clock a call came in. It was the matron of the local eventide home.

'I'm sorry to call so late but I'm worried about Mrs Donkin. Can't say what's wrong, but she won't take her tea.'

I felt this was a bit weak.

'How old is she, matron?'

'A hundred and twelve.'

'What did you say?' I gasped.

'I said a hundred and twelve,' she said impassively.

'I'll come at once.'

Eliza Donkin was indeed a hundred and twelve. Matron got so fed up with people doubting the fact that she had confirmed it with the parish register in Devon.

A bright-eyed old lady looked up at me like a little wizened bird. I listened to the ancient heart thudding in her shrivelled chest. A hand with crumpled tissue-paper skin and meandering blue veins reached out and pulled my arm. I bent over.

She whispered: 'Have you got a girl, young man? What about her?'

She pointed at the matron. She was about fifty-five and I was thirty-four – but from her vantage-point of years Mrs Donkin saw us both as youngsters, more or less of an age.

I smiled: 'I've got a girl already.'

She nodded happily.

In response to my companion's anxious but unspoken

question I said quietly, 'There's nothing definite, matron. Call me if there's any change.'

At half past eight she rang again.

'Mrs Donkin is unconscious. Could you come?'

As I hurried in, I could see she was very near the end. I listened again through the stethoscope: just four heartbeats and then silence.

I looked at the matron.

She sighed. 'In a month she would have been a hundred and thirteen. She's gone to glory instead.'

Back at the flat I stood looking out of the window. In the west, the sun had just dropped behind the hill. It had been a beautiful day.

Suddenly I thought of Fred's verse. I looked it up.

'There is a time to be born and a time to die.'

I thought of the morning's babe and Mrs Donkin's quiet departure; her time had been long in coming.

Fred might well be right in saying that you saw most things in this little town. Anyway, I'd seen the first and the last, in twenty-four hours.

4
Sic Transit . . .

I looked up from the newspaper.

'I wonder if sport influences your character and your career.' I knew it was an unoriginal thought but then I often have them. 'Here's Judge Aarvold sending some swindler down for a stretch. I remember Aarvold when he was a wing three-quarter captaining England against the Springboks.'

Elisabeth said, 'I'd say, it all depends and I wish you wouldn't put your feet on the sofa, I've just washed the covers.' I took them off.

'What d'you mean – it all depends? All depends on what?'

'Well, I suppose some sports could get you on the old-boy network; I haven't heard of many boxers becoming famous musicians though,' she added obliquely.

I said, 'No, but there are lots of rugger players who have become parsons.'

'So what?' said Elisabeth.

That seemed to be that, but I went on thinking about it on my rounds. Take Fred for instance. Gentle, fond of the exotic blooms in his greenhouse. He'd been a keen hockey player and my impressions of hockey – chiefly of the mixed variety – were of a fairly ferocious occupation; that wasn't Fred at all.

Then there was Charles: admittedly he had the shoulders and hands of a rowing blue, but he'd been a classics scholar before he'd turned to medicine and although he didn't suffer fools gladly, I reckoned him a jolly good doctor. Had rowing moulded him at all? Of course, his classics had given him a pretty mean start in medicine, where most of the terminology is based on Latin and Greek. I felt it - especially as my mediocre mind could only just cope with Cambridge Entrance Latin and Charles had the habit of summing up most situations with a classical quotation, few of which I understood.

And then there was me, what had rugby done to me?

I was still pondering the matter when I got back home for elevenses. There was Charles just coming out of a house opposite.

'Come in and have a coffee,' I called over.

When we were sitting drinking it, I asked him, 'Do you think sport moulds your personality?'

He put down his cup and a faraway look came into his eyes.

'Rowing – yes, that gives you concentration, precision, co-ordination. But rugby . . .'

I stopped him in mid-sentence, fearing another incomprehensible Greek quotation. 'Be honest Charles! You just hadn't the stomach for elemental physical contact.'

He looked at me and I felt suddenly conscious of my broken nose and cauliflower ears.

'You could be right,' he said.

'I don't mean you have to be a belligerent type,' I went on, 'though I did get a certain reputation among the sports writers – largely unwarranted – for being a rough player. But you know what a gentle chap I am by nature.'

Charles choked suddenly over his coffee. He put his cup down and said with his usual urbanity, 'I wonder what gave them that idea?'

I shrugged my shoulders. 'Howard Marshall usually gave me a good write-up in the *Telegraph*, but even he once said "Hamilton could qualify as a hand-to-hand fighter in the Abyssinian Army". Pure libel! But that sort of thing gets around. Before you know it, you're stuck with it. Elisabeth was once waiting in a queue at Twickenham and a chap in front said to his companion, "You know that chap Hamilton – he's the dirtiest player on the field and he teaches in a Sunday school".'

Charles had a second fit of coughing. When he had recovered I went on: 'I will admit I played vigorously, but I only punched a chap once and apologized immediately afterwards. He thought I was nuts! Hospital matches were really tough, as you know. When we were in Kenya, I took Elisabeth to a dentist in the local township. He looked at her name and asked if she happened to be related to Andy Hamilton. She said, "Yes, he's my husband. Why, have you met him?" "*Met him*?" His voice rose to a frenzied squeak, then he pulled up his trouser-leg and showed her a scar. "See that? That's where he tackled me in the Hospitals' Cup Match." But he didn't bear any malice, and did a good job on her tooth.'

Charles didn't think it necessary to comment. 'Did you play any rugger in Africa?' he asked instead.

'Yes, occasionally. But I had to play in plimsolls – takkies they call them out there; you see, I left my boots in England.'

'Just as well,' said Charles. I ignored this.

'A curious thing happened recently,' I continued. 'You remember that game I played for Sussex against the army a few weeks ago?'

'Yes, you scored a try, I hear.'

'Well, there was a chap in the Sussex team who apparently played with me in Kenya, though I didn't know it until my nephew in Nairobi sent me a newspaper cutting. It's in my writing desk.' I got it out. 'It says: "Never underestimate a Scot in takkies. There was a time when Nairobi arrived with only fourteen of the team. After considerable discussion among the elders it was announced, 'We've got a Soutie here with his takkies. We can't understand him – you're welcome man.'

"A missionary doctor, he had hitched in from the bottom of the escarpment but the locals were not very interested. They were after the game – he played a blinder for Nairobi. They were even more interested the next year and sent a congratulatory telegram when he was selected to play for Scotland again, having played nine times previously, pre-war." This chap went on: "One of my last matches before setting out again for Kenya was against the British Army and I was told they were to be skippered by a missionary doctor who was likely to be upset by my normal changing-room antics and that I really ought to curb myself. This was the case and I was somewhat apprehensive as to how this would affect the team's attitude on the field. I need not have worried, for this genteel Scot was transformed into a raging monster as soon as the whistle blew." '

Neither Charles nor Fred had raised any objection to my playing rugby on my free Saturdays so I had joined the Wilverton Club whose members included dentists, doctors, policemen, farmers, schoolmasters and servicemen on leave.

It wasn't long before we had a visit from a French team from Normandy who were on tour. They were very young, and the scrum-half was positively minute. In our second row was Police Sergeant Jones who hailed from South Wales. Mid-way through the second half there came a sudden deafening blast on the whistle. Jones stopped in his tracks; he was carrying the French half, ball and all, in a burst for the line.

'Put him down at once!' yelled the referee and added, *sotto voce*, '*C'est magnifique, mais ce n'est pas le rugby.*'

Our captain, a dentist, had sprained his wrist on a tough

31

molar, so I was acting-captain. When the score was 27–0 in our favour I said to the team, 'For goodness' sake chuck the ball about a bit.'

We did just that and a neat interception by the French centre ended in a try, so they went home with honour upheld and the *entente cordiale* only slightly dented.

It was easier to be called from the rugby field than from a sailing boat offshore, and the next weekend I was on second call for emergencies as Charles was out sailing. He had taken this up as the next best thing to rowing. We were in the early stages of the game when I noticed frantic signs from the girlfriend of one of our team which brought me off the field.

'Your partner Dr Wilson is out on an emergency. His wife says you're wanted at No. 75 on the front, Flat 4. It's a Mrs Saville and they think she has appendicitis. It sounded urgent.'

I trotted to the changing room, washed my hands and put on a raincoat – fortunately a long one – and drove straight to No. 75. It was about three-quarters of a mile away. The young husband was looking worried as he showed me into the bedroom. 'Glad you came so quickly, doctor. I think she's bad.'

Mrs Saville really was in pain. She lay curled up in the bed, white-faced, her tummy acutely tender down the right side and hard as a board. She had a slight rise in temperature and she had vomited. She hadn't had her bowels open since the day before. Everything was pointing to an acute appendicitis. When I had done a full examination I rose to my feet and my coat split open showing my muddy knees and rugger shorts.

'I feel she's got an acute appendix and needs admission to the Duke of Gloucester,' I said to Mr Saville. We got on the phone and the ambulance arrived in a few minutes.

When I rang the hospital that evening, the sister told me that Mrs Saville had had the op and they'd found an appendix on the point of bursting. A week later she was back home, well and convalescing.

I got one of those rare letters of thanks from Mr Saville. On the back of the letter he had done a marvellous cartoon of a lady in bed and over her was bending a figure with a stethoscope, wearing a scrum cap and dressed in rugger shirt, shorts, stockings and boots, with a cloud of steam rising from him. Saville was a commercial artist. That picture has a place of honour in my rugger photo album.

If letters of thanks were scarce, gifts were even scarcer – but they were much more of a problem. We were scared stiff of anything which might imply that we were giving preferential treatment to one person rather than another. Even the smallest legacies might suggest undue attention, but the most touching gifts were often the least deserved.

Miss Bracegirdle's was one of these. Miss Bracegirdle was a diabetic of limited means who had learned over the years the total management of her condition. She could adjust her insulin injections to a nicety without calling a doctor, but she had developed skin trouble and this necessitated several visits. At the end of these this gallant, independent old lady very shyly slipped a little tissue-paper parcel into my hand.

'That's for baby Barnaby,' she said. (She took a fervent interest in all our children.)

Quite overcome with surprise and pleasure I unwrapped a beautiful little silver trinket with a whistle in one end and silver bells hanging from the other, all suspended from a yellowing ivory ring. I'm no connoisseur of antiques but I recognized a really valuable early Victorian chewing ring and rattle.

'You really mustn't give me this, Miss Bracegirdle,' I protested. 'It's most valuable and if you knew Barnaby, you would realize that his mighty fists will destroy it in a minute.'

'Never mind, my dear doctor. I had it as a baby, and an old lady of eighty hasn't any more teeth to cut on it!' she chuckled. 'It will give me great pleasure if you'll take it.'

It's extraordinary how things happen in pairs.

That afternoon a very wealthy patient died at ninety-two. I paid my usual visit to offer comfort to the relatives and to give the death certificate. She had been a rather exacting patient and had always been visited regularly, but of recent months she had required visiting almost every day.

I was still feeling rather elevated by my morning gift of an antique silver rattle so when the old lady's daughter said to me 'There's a little packet left for you on the sideboard', I was quite overcome.

Surely the old lady hadn't sent out her housekeeper at the end of her life just to get a present for her doctor. The words 'But I really haven't done anything to deserve this' were almost on my lips as I unwrapped the parcel. Two pairs of rubber gloves and a half-used carton of glycerine suppositories were revealed. The words died in my throat. I went dumbly down the stairs.

With my duties, I could turn out only occasionally to play rugby for Wilverton. I wasn't really fit, so after a time, I filled in only when there was a vacancy. This Saturday, I was playing at full-back for the Extra A team where I didn't have to run much. I had hoped to keep going until I could play one game with Peter, who was showing promise, even at his tender age.

The opposing wing three-quarter broke away and I summoned up just enough energy to bring him down before he scored. As we fell together, I felt a crunching pain in my left hip.

In the bath afterwards it began to feel better. I lay back and thought of other games. There is nothing like exhaustion and hot water for conjuring up nostalgic memories. Two especially stood out: One of Twickenham, one of Murrayfield. Oddly enough, Africa was linked with both.

Because of the Twickenham match, my whole future might have changed. It was like this. When the war came, I gave up all hope of medical missionary work and made enquiries about entry into the Parachute Regiment. I was nearing the end of my hospital job and was considered safe to be loosed on the unsuspecting British soldiery. I had in fact made a brief attempt to investigate the possibility of serving abroad in the Colonial Medical Service. It had been amusing but abortive.

My interview was at 2.30 p.m. on a Monday at their offices in Queen Anne's Gate. At 2.15 I turned up at the imposing building. I was dressed in my one good suit. I waited half an hour in the mahogany-panelled library. A harassed-looking clerk came in bearing a folder.

'I'm sorry Dr Hamilton, we have no news yet of your passage to Penang.' He looked at me apprehensively over his gold-rimmed specs.

'I haven't come for a passage, only for an interview.'

He pushed up his glasses and looked down at the folder. 'You are Dr Andrew Hamilton?'

'Yes, but this is the first contact I have had with the Colonial Medical Service.'

He started and peered at me again over his glasses. 'Oh dear, I am so sorry! I see you are not forty years of age.' He giggled rather weakly. 'There must be another Dr Andrew Hamilton.'

There was; I knew there was. A few weeks before I had received a threatening letter from a firm of money-lenders demanding repayment of £200, and I guessed I had a some-what profligate namesake.

I still had a slight feeling of confusion when, at last, I was ushered into the 'Presence'. The Secretary was a grey-haired man who had the aloofness befitting one so exalted. I got off to a bad start.

'Why do you want to join the Service, Dr Hamilton?' His tone implied my seeking membership of a very exclusive club.

'Well sir, I always planned to do medical missionary work. As this is not possible at present, I felt I might still serve the country abroad in the Colonial Medical Service.'

This was honest but hardly tactful. Outrage showed all over his face. Here was a would-be missionary applying *as second choice* to the one, the august, the ultimate medical work overseas, the Colonial Medical Service! I suppose I'd asked for it and I got a right going-over, but after five minutes I began to seethe with indignation. After all, all I'd come for was information, not a catechizing.

Finally he said, 'Well, that will be all, doctor.'

I rose to go and was turning to the door when he said, 'By the way, do you play any sport?'

I thought, 'This is my turn', and answered quietly, 'I have played rugby for Scotland.'

I glanced at his face. The transformation was remarkable. His eyebrows descended to a normal level. He swallowed and when he spoke it was in honeyed tones.

'My dear fellow – of course. I thought I knew your name. I watched you at Twickers in the Calcutta Cup in 1938. Why didn't you mention it?'

'You didn't ask me,' I answered coolly.

'Then may I say, you are *just* the type we are looking for in the Service. Keen on sport, able to cope with tough situations. We would welcome your application. In fact the Sudan is needing medical officers right now. If you want to proceed further, please get in touch directly with me. Goodbye now, goodbye, delighted to have met you.' He leaned forward and shook my hand – for the first time.

I managed not to laugh until I was halfway down the stairs. As I walked out into the fuss and throb of London traffic, I pictured him going to his club that evening. 'Interesting chap came for an interview today. Hamilton, you know, Scottish international, played nine times in a row; was in the side that got the Triple Crown at Twickenham before the king. Good chap – hope he applies.'

As I was sauntering along Whitehall, I thought how curious it is that sport's valued so highly. He hadn't asked much about my degrees or experience.

I decided against the Colonial Medical Service – and yet, when I was in Africa, I did find that rugger had not been a total waste of time. I'd learned to keep on despite utter exhaustion and accept defeat as part of the game. I found too, that the mountain tribesmen of Kenya were natural athletes beyond compare and that their trackless wilderness demanded the ultimate in physical fitness. Perhaps that Secretary had a point. Colonial officials, now so much maligned, did their job with a determined sense of fair play, even without a referee's whistle.

The other game – the Murrayfield one – that came to mind as I lay in steaming languor was my very last for Scotland. It was after our voyage home on our first leave from Africa.

36

I'd been wondering if I could possibly get back in the team after so many years. Was there a chance? Well, I would jolly well get fit and have a go, so I started training on board ship.

I had just completed ten circuits of the deck and the sun was sinking in the Red Sea, when a fellow passenger called from his deck-chair, 'What on earth are you doing, Andrew? Isn't it hot enough for you?'

'Fitness my lad,' I gasped, 'fitness,' as the sweat ran off me in rivulets. 'You should try it sometime.'

He laughed and finished his beer.

I kept it up all the way to Plymouth.

Elisabeth wasn't very well and this and the children kept our hands full until January, then I joined the London Scottish and was given a game in the A team. I found to my great satisfaction that living at 8,000 feet in Kenya seemed to have boosted my red blood supply to enable me to utilize the rarefied atmospheric oxygen more efficiently, and so I had plenty of wind at sea level.

Next game, I was transferred to the First XV. All the Scottish trial matches were over and naturally I had not been able to play in any of them, but a selector was watching this game, I was told afterwards.

Scotland, sadly, were beaten by both Wales and Ireland and the selectors were scraping the barrel for players, and so it seems they came on me down there at the bottom, the sole survivor of that side that got the Triple Crown. They picked me for the match against England.

As we laced our boots in the changing-room we could hear the stamp and roar of the crowd in the stands overhead, and the noise made all our hearts beat faster. I prayed a short silent prayer: 'Let me play this game for you, Lord.' As I thought of those pre-war games, it seemed that I'd played them very much for my own glory and I wanted this one, my last, to be different.

The selector who'd watched me with the London Scottish came into the room.

'Don't let me down, Andy,' he whispered, and I guessed that it was he who had suggested to the other selectors that there was life in the old dog yet, at nearly thirty-three.

It was a ding-dong game and time was running out with England just in the lead. I wasn't running madly everywhere this time as I had done in the past before the war, but I was conserving my energy for the critical moments. I needed to – energy was in rather short supply.

At last the ball went into touch twenty yards from the English line, down at the left-hand corner. The throw-in wasn't a good one, and the ball bounced off several desperately clutching hands before it dropped into mine at the back of the line-out. I went for the line. There was a phalanx of muddy white jerseys in the way, but I jinked and twisted and broke through to the full-back. As he went for my knees I handed him off fiercely into the mud, and with several sets of fingers clutching the back of my shorts I dived for the line.

The ball thumped down in my outstretched hands and the whistle went. When I picked it up, the ball had a white patch on it where it had hit the chalk. I threw it back to the goal-kicker and inside I said, 'Thank you'. That try beat England.

A day or two later I'd had a letter from a retired missionary doctor in Scotland. He wrote to me and I could still almost imagine him saying it: 'I was listening on the wireless and when I heard you'd scored I could-na help mesel' shouting "P-r-r-aise the Lor-r-d!"'

'Hear! Hear!' I'd felt like saying.

I got out of the bath and as I cooled off, the pain in my hip came back. 'That's my lot,' I said to myself. 'This is my last game.'

I even managed to emulate Charles by mentally concocting a Latin tag for the occasion: *Sic transit gloria rugbyi*, which freely translated would mean I guess, 'Old rugby players never die, they simply keep on talking about the past!'

5
Still waters

The three of us were standing in Fred's consulting-room: we all opened our eyes, raised our heads and the other two began getting about their business. I just stood there. In the practice, we always began the day with a few minutes of prayer together before the rush started. We felt that after this, we'd be more inclined to give the patients an even break and less likely to get steamed up with one another over trifles.

It usually worked very well but I wasn't with it today. I'd been turning over a grievance in my mind ever since I'd got in and I'd got to get it off my chest somehow. Miss Spencer had decamped to let in the impatient hordes and Fred was sitting down, going through some records. I let go.

'Fred,' my voice sounded unpleasantly high-pitched. 'Fred, I know it's not a good time but I have a small bone to pick.'

Fred looked up mildly: 'Sorry about that Andy, what's the difficulty?'

I knew it was going to sound pathetic but I plugged on.

'Well, I can't help noticing that I seem to be getting the heavy end of the visiting lately.'

'You mean you're getting more than your share of new visits in the surgery book? Well, we can soon sort it out. Have you got your own book Andy?'

I produced it and put it by his on the desk. When I compared them, day by day, it was quite obvious that if anybody had got the heavy end, it was Fred not me.

'You see,' Fred said patiently, 'I don't want too many of my old folks having to send for me so when I call, I tell them when I'm going to make the next visit and book it down ahead. That saves them worrying and it spreads the load for me too.'

I hung my head. 'Sorry, Fred.'

'Not to worry Andy, best to get things in the clear.'

I was beginning to realize there was a lot about Fred I didn't know yet. Good things I envied. Not that he never put a foot wrong, though.

When I saw one of his more difficult patients' cards on my desk one morning, I felt a nasty twinge of apprehension about the midriff region. She was an aged, dowager-duchess type who had gradually created a neutral zone around herself by her austere approach and, friendless, had developed an interesting series of psychosomatic ailments to compensate.

She made etiquette of small account by announcing before she had barely seated herself, 'I saw your colleague Wilson last week about my migraine, and I have no wish to see him again. He had the impertinence to imply that my disability was due to loneliness and he asked me if I belonged to a church. I replied, "Indeed I do, *young* man," (Fred had topped fifty), "and have done for seventy years. Do you?" '

Something else hitherto unsuspected (by me) about Fred's make-up came to light one day, the week after my morning moan in the surgery. I had an unexpected spring-clean to do – on the ear of a chap who'd broken his femur in a car accident and couldn't hear his bedside radio. As his house was quite near Fred's, I popped to see if he had a spare ear-syringe to lend. Grace produced a magnificent brass weapon, of obvious fire-power, for me.

'This is the one he used on the Jap commandant,' she informed me. 'That was when I thought Fred was going to be shot,' she added.

'I can quite understand that!' I said, weighing the monster cylinder in my hand.

'No, I don't mean it like that,' said Grace.

They had both been in China doing hospital work during the war; their area had been overrun by the Japanese and they were interned in their own hospital.

'The food was appalling,' she went on, 'and the children were going down like flies with malnutrition, so Fred told the commandant that he wouldn't treat any more Jap soldiers unless the children's rations were improved. He was marched off and I thought that was the last time I would see him alive, but he came back smiling and the children's food became much better.'

But it wasn't until little Figley's court appearance came up that Fred's real quality was revealed to me. It had seemed an open and shut case. Figley was a pathetic little man with a scatty, extravagant wife and two wild teenage kids. He had gone to Wilverton's biggest multiple store, paid for some groceries and just walked out with several pairs of woollen socks under his arm. He'd only gone twenty-five yards before being stopped by the store detective.

Apparently Figley said that he had an awful headache and hadn't known what he was doing, but the store manager had been losing so much stock that he was out for blood. I guessed his job was in danger. He called the police and preferred charges, even though the stuff was only worth a quid or two. Poor Figley was cautioned, questioned and charged and in due course he was to appear in court.

His wife came and begged Fred to say something in her husband's favour. Fred quite rightly told her to get legal aid and a solicitor, and he gave her the name of a good one. Next, Fred was asked for a medical report and later to appear in court to give evidence for the defence. On the day of the trial, I was determined to get through my visits and be there, if I possibly could, to hear Fred in the witness-box. This was one occasion I was not going to miss.

As luck would have it, it was one of those occasional slack days and there were only three visits in the book for me. The first was a poor little girl with a bad ear. I gave her an injection of penicillin, very regretfully, for the poor mite was sobbing with the pain in her ear and I had to add another one in her bottom.

Next, I went on to a damp basement to treat a coalman with bronchitis. He, poor man, had given up the unequal struggle against coal-dust and, in the dim light of the basement, his face and hands were only distinguishable from the sheet and pillow-case by being just one shade blacker. I made a note to get the welfare and the Medical Officer of Health onto his case and set off, en route for my last case.

A neighbour had sent in a message saying, 'Could the

doctor call on Mrs Bigworth as she was proper poorly and had been for weeks, only she wouldn't send herself'. It might be something or nothing, we would have to see.

I hurried up the path to the front door. There was a painter on a ladder propped across it. As I edged underneath, a cheerful voice said, 'Mornin', doc.'

I found myself looking up into a sunburnt face, grinning down at me. He, no doubt, had seen the ends of my stethoscope sticking out of my coat pocket. 'Good morning,' I answered hurriedly.

The door of Mrs Bigworth's flat was ajar. I knocked and walked in. She was sitting in a chair by the fire. At once, I noticed her peculiar colour.

I greeted her and then I said, 'Mrs Bigworth, I wonder if you would mind turning your face to the window?' As she did so, I saw that her skin had indeed a peculiar lemon-yellow tint.

I examined her tongue. It looked like raw meat.

'How are you feeling these days?' I asked.

'Poorly, doctor, least bit of work makes me breathless and gives me a tight pain across my chest.'

'How do you feel on your pins?'

'Funny you should ask about my feet, doctor; they really are most peculiar, all pins and needly and when I walk, it's like walking on rubber balloons – can't feel the floor under them.'

I tapped her Achilles tendons; there was practically no response and she had lost a lot of sensation too. I had no doubt about it now. She had pernicious anaemia and must have had it for some time as she was now developing nerve involvement as well. I sat down.

'Mrs Bigworth, you have got a certain kind of anaemia. I'm pretty sure, but I will need to take a blood test to confirm it.'

'Is it bad, doctor?'

'No, only if you don't get it treated. You *were* naughty, you know, you should have sent before.'

'But we don't like to bother you doctors, you've got folks much worse than me.'

42

'You're a patient too, Mrs Bigworth, and you're not calling us unnecessarily.'

I boiled up a syringe – no pre-packed, sterile, throw-away models then – and took her blood.

'Does it look a good colour, doctor?' she asked.

'You can't tell by looking at it. I'll have to get it tested in the lab. So, goodbye for now, I'll be back and I'm sure we can get you right and keep you right, but it will mean having injections, maybe for the rest of your life.'

I looked at my watch on the way out. Figley's case would be starting in about an hour and I'd got to get this blood to the lab. I wasn't too pleased when I found the painter on the step waiting for me.

'I like the look of you, doc. Take me on your books will you? I haven't registered with anyone yet, not long come out of the forces.'

'I expect we can arrange that,' I answered briskly, thinking that my lunch prospect was fast disappearing over the horizon. 'Where do you live?'

'Payne Hill, and the name is Hodd, Bert Hodd.'

'That's OK,' I said. 'Send in your card and we'll take you. I bet you don't ail much – just the sort of patient we like!'

He laughed. Then, and I really should have kept my mouth shut if I wanted to get to that court in time, I asked, 'Where were you serving?'

'Tank Corps, Middle East. Early on, I was with Monty in the desert campaign. Funny, had to do a job for the medical officer there once. Told me to take a section and collect a body that had been washed up on the shore of the Med. Poor RAF bloke who'd been shot down. Found out who he was too – Lord David Douglas-Hamilton.'

I swallowed but said nothing for a moment or two. My mind was going back to an uproarious dinner at Cambridge in 1936 after the university boxing match, and the tall, darkly handsome man who had sat opposite me. He should have been my opponent as the Oxford heavyweight. But he'd been unable to train for the bout because of exams. I beat de Villiers Graaf, who took his place. But if it had been that tall, dark man – well, the result would have been different, for he was David Douglas-Hamilton, a brilliant boxer. I found he was charmingly modest as well. I thought sadly of him now, buried in the sands of North Africa. Then I suddenly came to. I would have to miss lunch if I was going to get to that court on time.

I rang Elizabeth from a call-box and went on to the hospital with my specimen of blood . . . I ran up the steps of the courthouse and crept in at the back. Then I discovered that the earlier cases had obviously taken less time than expected and Mr Uffington-Bragg was just rising to cross-examine Fred who had become the star witness for the defence and had already given his evidence.

The thing was that little Figley really *did* have a defence. He was quite a severe diabetic. Uffington-Bragg was a huge man with bulging paunch and bristling side-whiskers.

'Now, doctor,' he began. 'You said in your evidence as the accused's physician, that, in your opinion his admitted taking of goods, without paying for them, could have been due to a state of mind induced by an attack of acute hyperglycaemia. . .'

Before he could pursue his questioning, Fred broke in with unexpected temerity, 'Do you not mean hypoglycaemia?'

Uffington-Bragg swelled visibly before replying in awesome tones, 'Sir, in this court it is not your prerogative to *ask* questions, it is your duty to *answer* them.'

Fred looked calmly across the court, but I caught a metallic glint behind his glasses.

'I do apologize, I was simply trying to be helpful. You see, if you do not know what you are talking about, you are unlikely to get the answers you require.'

The chairman of the bench quickly put his hand up in front of his mouth while Uffington-Bragg stood there with his eyes popping out and his mouth opening and shutting like a landed cod, without uttering a sound.

'You really must not speak to the prosecuting solicitor like that, Dr Wilson,' said the chairman.

'I do apologize,' said Fred again.

The chairman turned to Uffington-Bragg who was shuffling his papers with a midnight scowl on his face. 'Please continue your cross-examination.'

I have no more questions for this witness,' said Uffington-Bragg, in a voice suggesting the sound of gas escaping from a pricked balloon.

I had to leave at that point but I laughed all the way to the car at the way dear, mild Fred had accomplished the demolition of that bombastic bully. Charles and I heard the sequel from Fred's own lips the following morning.

'Glad to say, little Figley got off. But, when I was leaving the court, an usher came up and said that Mr Entwhistle, the chairman, wanted to see me in the retiring room, if I could spare the time. He got up as I went in, shook my hand and offered me a cup of tea. You know we were up at Oxford together? Funnily enough so was Uffington-Bragg. Entwhistle said, "I wanted to congratulate you on the way you put down old Puffy-Bragg. I've been longing to do that for ages but have never got the chance! Poor old chap, he never could get his Greek prefixes right." '

Two days later, I got the result of the blood test back from the lab. She'd got pernicious anaemia all right: the specimen was full of typical immature large blood cells. I showed the report to Fred.

'I suggest you explain to her simply what is wrong and then she'll be willing to continue the injections even after she feels better.'

I told Fred about Bert Hodd the painter. 'Ask him if he'd like to do the outside of our house, if you see him,' he said. Bert was still there doing the windows so I gave him the message.

I explained to Mrs Bigworth that her stomach had stopped making a chemical which was necessary to combine with her food to enable her body to make proper blood cells, and we would have to go on giving her that chemical, by injection, to keep things right. She understood very well and I gave her the first injection of cyanocobalamin, the chemical in question, thankful that years of medical detective work and research had made this hitherto sinister condition so easily

45

treatable. A pound or two of raw liver daily had been the old remedy!

Two months later, she walked gaily into the surgery for her next injection and, around the same time, Fred told me that his house was now looking, as Bert Hodd put it, 'a treat'.

6
The Semple touch

Charles meant it when he promised to help me get the hang of general practice. We didn't have formal teaching sessions. I had to pick it up as I went along, mostly by listening to his throw-away lines. 'When they call you – you go'. 'Examine the patient first, save your tick-off till after. You may not feel like it then.' But I learnt the hard way.

I reacted so quickly at night to the telephone that I would have the receiver to my ear before the bell rang twice. This doesn't mean I felt any better about being disturbed.

'Doctor Hamilton, can you come and see the baby? He won't stop crying. I don't know what's the matter with him.'

'What's your name?'

'Mrs James. I live at 49 Jarvis Lane.'

'All right, I'll be along.'

I had to turn on the bedside light to see my way around. I glanced at the clock. It was 3 a.m. Elisabeth said sleepily, 'I'm sorry you've got to go out Andy', and turned over.

As I drove to the council estate up on the edge of the Downs I was thinking, 'I don't wish anybody ill but I hope this is a necessary call.' It was that time of the night when you feel at your worst. You're getting nicely down to the business of sleeping when you are jerked out by the scruff of your neck, and sent off to solve the minor whodunnit of another case.

Mrs James led me into the bedroom. Her baby was crying lustily. I examined him thoroughly and I could find nothing wrong. Then I undid his nappies and a strong smell of ammonia hit me in the nostrils. He kicked and screamed. His nappy was soaking, and he had a brilliant red rash around his bottom.

'Look at this, Mrs James. This is what's wrong. You haven't been looking after this baby properly and you've called me out in the night for a nappy rash.'

I stopped suddenly. Why didn't I remember Charles's advice? Mrs James was crying and I felt bad.

'Doctor,' she sobbed, 'I'm sorry, it wasn't just the baby I wanted you for. It was my husband. When the baby cried, he got up quick and then he fell all of a heap and kicked around on the floor. My dad came in and when Jim came to, he wanted to fight him.'

I began to feel a proper heel.

'Where is he, Mrs James?'

'Next room, doctor. He seems all funny.'

I went through. The man was lying on the bed snoring. I shook him gently. He slowly came round and when I asked him questions, his answers were all fuddled. When I got the story straight it was pretty obvious what the trouble was. He had had his first epileptic fit. In the long run, it turned out that he was to have many more before we got his medication right.

I went back to Mrs James. 'I'm very sorry. Perhaps if you'd told me first about your husband. . .'

'It's all right, doctor. I'm sorry too.'

'Now listen. I've given your husband a tablet for tonight. He'd better come to see someone in the morning.'

I packed up and went home.

I woke late next morning and got to the surgery after the morning session had started. I was due for visiting anyway. I was writing out my list when the surgery door was flung open and a lady with a shopping basket came dashing in.

'Doctor, can you come round the corner please? There's an old lady lying in the road.'

I called Charles and he felt it was something he'd better handle.

'You might as well come too though,' he said. 'You might learn something, you never know.'

We walked about a hundred yards up the road and ahead of us we could see a small crowd. They were gathered round an old lady who was lying in the gutter. We pushed through and then Charles whispered to me, 'It's our Miss Cramp.'

She lay there with her eyes open and a faint smile on her lips. A young man in a sports jacket was bending over her. I caught his eyes for a moment and there was a professional gleam in them. When he saw us he straightened up.

'What's happened?' Charles asked briskly.

'I'm a medical student,' the young man said, with dignity. 'I think she's knocked her head and is suffering from post traumatic retrograde amnesia. I can't get anything out of her.'

Charles looked down at Miss Cramp.

'No,' he said. 'That's because she's nearly stone deaf.'

He bent down and put one arm under Miss Cramp's shoulder and lifted her gently into a sitting position.

She smiled at him. 'Ah, Doctor Semple. I slipped off the curb and fell. I couldn't get up again. But do you know I'm perfectly certain it was a firecrest I saw in the hedge. They're very uncommon here.'

Miss Cramp, though very deaf, was an ardent ornithologist.

Charles never wasted time or words. He smiled at Miss Cramp, then he bent and bellowed in her ear. 'You must record it when you get home. Do you think you can get up?'

With my help and that of the student – now a much chastened individual – Charles got Miss Cramp to her feet and we escorted her to the surgery. She was drinking a cup of tea when I set out on my belated round of visits.

I went to the first address on my list. No one came in answer to the ring, but through the door I could hear a ferocious barking. I tried the handle and found that the door would open. The call hadn't specified what was wrong and

I had visions of someone very ill and the only help at hand a faithful dog.

I opened the door a few inches. Inside, two large black Alsatians were bounding around the small entrance hall. They were barking their heads off, and snarling with bared teeth. I shut the door again very quickly. What on earth was I going to do? Perhaps Mrs Hickes was upstairs, too ill to call off the dogs. I must get in and attend to her.

I remembered another of Charles's words of wisdom: 'Don't fraternize with patients' dogs.' It would have been wise to follow his advice now, but I was feeling mildly heroic and I wasn't aiming to do any fraternization anyway, only to get in.

I pushed the door open suddenly and warded off the slavering hounds with my visiting bag as I retreated backwards up the stairs. Fortunately, the dogs had evidently been trained to stay downstairs so they didn't pursue me, but my bag will bear the marks of their teeth for many a day. I knocked on the doors of all three bedrooms in turn. There was no reply so I walked into them one after another.

There was nobody in the house. My spirit of devotion and self-sacrifice evaporated rapidly, leaving me with a feeling which was a mixture of fear and rage. Here was I, besieged by a pair of bloodthirsty black hounds, and there was no wretched patient anyway.

While I was contemplating how to make my escape the front door opened and the ferocious beasts suddenly became a pair of slobbering acolytes, fawning on their mistress.

'Oh hullo, doctor,' she called up cheerily. 'Sorry not to be in. I felt a lot better so I popped out for some cigarettes. I didn't expect you so early.'

I descended the stairs with dignity.

'Mrs Hickes. I would just like to make two points. First, if you were well enough to go shopping, you were well enough to come to the surgery and in any case you could have cancelled my visit. Second, I do not expect, when visiting a patient, to be savaged by a pair of ferocious dogs. If you really need my help, you can come to the surgery. Good morning.'

I had recovered by the time I was bumping up a rutted, unmade road to my next port of call. It was an old, red-brick house which looked like several farm labourers' cottages knocked into one. The outside of the house was shabby, but it was nothing to the state of affairs inside.

African huts may have been primitive but they were always swept out daily with a bunch of aromatic bushes, and the blankets and sleeping-skins put out in the morning sun to discourage bed bugs. This house, in an English coastal resort, beat them into a cocked hat. Three storeys high, it had three main rooms on each floor. Four families shared it with at least ten children amongst them, not to mention assorted dogs and cats.

I was to see a baby with a cough. A rather bedraggled family greeted me at the door and led me into the living-room. The poor little unwashed mite was lying in a pram tucked beside an open fireplace. The room was filthy. I think there was lino on the floor but I couldn't be certain because my shoes slid on a quarter-inch thick matting of sticky dirt.

A connecting door led through to the kitchen. I saw a greasy gas stove in one corner and a sink with a cold tap alongside. There was a heap of coal just lying in another corner. Across the centre of the cement floor an open drain from the sink ran to an outlet in the wall. The living-room wall had a crack in the plaster large enough for me to put my fist in, and I could see daylight on the far side.

I lifted the crying child from the pram and, with half a dozen other grubby urchins gathered round, did my best to examine it. It didn't take long, for the reason for the cough was obvious. The poor little fellow was covered in a rash and his eyes were exuding pus. He had measles.

It was far too late to try to isolate the child. I gave the mother instructions on how to nurse it, prescribed a liquid sulphonamide, eye drops and cough mixture and went off to arrange for a health visitor to call to supervise its care.

When I told Charles about it, his reply was as succinct as always: 'It's a case for the Medical Officer of Health.'

Next morning Charles gave me a progress report.

'I saw old Macfarlane. He didn't seem very concerned.

"It would have to be investigated with gr-r-reat car-r-re. There is a big housing shor-r-tage" and all that. I discussed with him the advantages of putting the MP and the newspapers in the picture. This somehow seemed to inspire him. I think we shall get some action.'

He was right. In three weeks, all four families were rehoused. A little later, a wooden fence was put round the old house and the landlords were renovating it throughout.

But we were on the brink of a full-scale measles epidemic. Before we had been able to quarantine all the families in the red-brick house, they had spread the infection far and wide through several schools which the children attended.

It was a winter we would like to forget. Charles, Fred and I worked flat out. Measles was much more virulent then and the side-effects more frequent than in later years. The sulphonamide drugs and penicillin injections helped prevent the worst complications but, just when we were beginning to feel that the tide was turning, whooping cough broke out and the infant population took the brunt of it at the most vulnerable period of their lives.

Charles worked with amazing speed. He would finish his surgery when I was only half-way through mine. He would be home and dry from his visits by lunch-time while I was labouring on into the afternoon.

'Dr Semple, now there's a man for you,' said Mrs Sampson, an old stalwart of the practice. 'Knows what's wrong with you as soon as he comes in the door. So quick he is – meets himself coming out of the house when he's going in!'

Charles himself would say, 'If you haven't diagnosed your patient by the time he's sat down, you aren't much of a doctor.'

I took his words to heart.

One day, Elwyn Jenkins came in limping badly.

I said to myself with confidence, 'Retired Welsh miner, arthritic knees, secondary to years of kneeling at the coal seam. He'll be wanting analgesics and physiotherapy.'

'Come for my ears syringing haven't I, doctor. Can't even hear myself doing "Land of my Fathers" in the bath, isn't it?' he announced.

51

I felt in despair.

And I lost the practice a patient without even trying. It was the afternoon when the retired bank manager came in for an examination to test his fitness to drive.

'Just sign the paper here, young man,' he said.

I looked at the form. 'I certify that I have examined . . . and found that he has no condition which would render him unfit to drive, and I have informed the applicant accordingly.'

I glanced at his case notes and started. There was a report from an optician which stated, 'Very little sight in his right eye, 6/36, with correction in the left.'

'I'm sorry sir, but you appear to have deficient eyesight.' I glanced at him apologetically.

'Of course I haven't, young man. Are you refusing to sign that certificate?'

'I'm afraid I cannot sign it unless you are able to pass an eye test that I will give you, and also to satisfy me on examining you that you are fit to drive.'

I was getting a bit stroppy now as well.

'I've no intention of doing any such thing,' he said.

He grabbed the certificate, stood up and glared wildly round. 'Where's the door?' I took his arm and led him to it. That was the last we saw of him in our practice – but I suspect he's still driving around!

When I told Charles apologetically that we were one patient less he was reassuring.

'Andy, you needn't feel you've let us down. There was nothing else you could do. Anyway, we all lose patients. Did I tell you what happened to me when I was doing a locum before I came to this practice? My chief went on holiday and left me a list of visits which I must do as a routine. One of them was a very important, prize patient and she was to be given an injection of vitamins which I felt was a perfectly useless exercise.

'I arrived at the mansion, the door was opened by a butler and I was requested to wait in the hall. Eventually I was shown up into the bedroom and there, in a four-poster, was a fierce-looking dame who fixed me with her baleful eyes but did not speak. I gather she had had a stroke and lost all power of speech. I filled the syringe with the ghastly sticky stuff and pointed the needle upwards to expel the air. Unfortunately I didn't hold on to it, and ping, it shot off like an arrow and stuck in the ceiling and the vitamins were spread all over the room!

'I was at a loss for the moment, but then I turned to the old lady, still regarding me with an unwinking eye and expression of total disdain, and said, "Ah well, madam, it will do you no harm up there", patted her arm and left.

'My chief lost his patient and I lost the job. So never mind, Andy, you're in good company – mine!'

Viewing it objectively, I wouldn't say that modesty was Charles's most outstanding attribute.

7
Miss Spencer

I was in the little office reading the hospital reports that had come by second post the previous day. A few feet away sat Miss Spencer at the reception desk.

'Hullo Jimmy, what brings you here?'

I peeped surreptitiously into the waiting-room. A red-haired young man was standing there.

'Dropped a length of guttering on me foot, didn't I, Miss Spencer. Could I see Dr Semple d'you think?'

'Right-o, you'll be number six.'

She rose and came over to get his records from the files.

'One of my boys,' she whispered proudly.

She had been running a Sunday school class for as long as she'd been in the practice. This must be one of her earlier members.

'Always so clumsy,' she added affectionately. 'Now he's a

bricklayer I'm astonished he hasn't yet dropped one on somebody's head.'

This was the Spencer magic. She knew everybody, and most of them from childhood. How many mistakes and wasted journeys it saved us! I don't like being told what to do, but I grew to appreciate her advice, always offered very tactfully.

'I think it would be wise to put Mr Forsythe first on your list, doctor. His asthma can be very bad. Do you need any ampoules of adrenalin for your bag?' There's nothing worse than arriving at an unexpected asthma case and finding you've no injections. Broncho-dilator aerosols and steroid injections were still in the future; adrenalin had its dangers but usually it worked like a charm.

I was in the middle of giving Mr Wingate the second of his annual course of anti-catarrh injections in whose properties he had great faith (though I had my doubts), when I heard the noise start up in the waiting-room. I quickly swabbed his arm.

'Call in a week's time for the next, Mr Wingate. Would you see yourself out? I'm needed in the office.'

I darted across the tiled yard and whipped open the waiting-room door but Charles had got there first. A loud unpleasant voice assailed my ears.

'And just *who* do you think you are, telling me what I can and can't do! I demand to see a doctor at once. I can report you, you know!'

'Can I be of assistance?' I knew that steely note in Charles's voice. If I'd been the florid city gent harassing Miss Spencer, I would now have been taking evasive action. 'What seems to be the trouble?' Charles sounded positively silky.

'This wretched woman says the surgery is over, but you're here aren't you? I'm a busy man and I'm not being fobbed off like this.'

'Are you a patient of this practice then, Mr . . . er?'

'Barlow's the name. No, I'm not. My own doctor's on his day off and I require something for my indigestion.'

From the atmosphere in the waiting-room, I guessed that

54

over-indulgence in malt liquors was the likely cause of his malady.

I caught a glimpse of Miss Spencer, white-faced and trembling but still unflinching at her post, and I began to feel very angry. But Charles was moving quietly towards our visitor, so I kept in the background.

A hand, whose prehensile strength had been developed by being wrapped round many an oar, reached out and took the other's upper arm in a vice-like grip.

'My dear sir,' he was purring now, 'I do not think your medical requirements constitute an emergency, and what is more, you have been extremely offensive to our secretary, who is acting entirely on our instructions. I suggest you call on your own practitioner tomorrow morning during his surgery hours, if you still need advice. As you are leaving now, I wish you a very good night.'

The would-be patient was moving inexorably towards the door. As he reached it, his pace accelerated and he positively ran down the steps. To my utter astonishment, when he was in full flight, he meekly turned his head and murmured thickly, 'Good night to you.'

My partner closed the door softly and turned the key.

'Nice work, Charles,' I said under my breath, 'I wish I had your nerve.'

'Are you all right, Miss Spencer?' He was genuinely concerned. Her colour was coming back as she nodded. 'If our friend ever turns up again, just ring for one of us, won't you?' Charles concluded.

By no stretch of the imagination could Miss Spencer be described as a model secretary. Anyway, a 'model' may be defined as a small reproduction of the real thing, and Miss Spencer's functional capacity was larger than life.

Admittedly her filing system consisted of stocks of large labelled envelopes kept in a cupboard and her typing, of the one-finger variety, was highly individual. Nevertheless, letters went on time, bills were paid and tax-collectors kept at bay. She performed simple pathological tests, answered the telephone, acted as chaperone for lady patients, and she made the coffee. Moreover, she was a trained dispenser and although we were no longer a dispensing practice, her knowledge was invaluable when patients asked worried questions about their prescriptions. And in the old days, there was one of her specials – a mixture for nervous indigestion, prescribed under the shorthand title 'Mist. Spenceri'.

Miss Spencer really could almost have run the practice by herself. She nearly did during the war when she only had an old retired doctor to work with – as Dr Semple had been called up – but no one complained. They were probably too busy dodging bombs anyway by all accounts.

Miss Spencer lived about six miles out of town at Brendon, a pretty downland village, where she looked after her mother and brother in an old vicarage. Every day she drove to work in her battered Morris to open the surgery, promptly at 8.30. That is, every day but one.

I came at a quarter to nine and heard the banging on the waiting-room door from outside in the car park. When I opened it, I was nearly trampled underfoot by the rush for the reception desk. 'Where's Miss Spencer then?' our local butcher demanded, holding his bandaged thumb in his other hand.

Where was she indeed?

Fred arrived and we had a hurried conference in his surgery.

'Miss Spencer's not here.' I felt all at sea.

'Well, you man the reception desk and I'll start surgery. Perhaps she's got held up on the way here. She would have phoned if she was ill.'

There were about six people at the reception window all together. Miss Spencer would have never tolerated that.

'Now then, please make a line, and come one by one and tell me your names and addresses.'

'Miss Spencer knows who we are without being told.'

'Well, I don't, so please do as I say.'

I had just got out the fourth record-card when the phone rang.

'Surgery, can I help you?'

'That doctor's?' It was a broad Sussex voice. 'D'you 'ave

a lady, name of Spencer, workin' for ye? Wants a word, she does. 'Ere Missus, speak to 'em yerself.'

'Doctor? Oh Doctor Hamilton, I'm so sorry. I'm afraid I am going to be late. There's been a slight accident with my car.' Her voice wavered a little as she finished.

'Miss Spencer, please, are you all right, tell me?' I was gabbling with anxiety. 'What has happened? Where are you?'

Her voice came back, controlled and soothing. 'Now doctor, don't get upset. You are not to worry, I am quite all right.' She sounded exactly as she did when comforting a child afraid of having an injection. 'But I'm afraid my car won't get me to the surgery.'

'Where *are* you, Miss Spencer? I *am* worried.'

'I'm safe and sound in a cottage, half-way down Brendon Hill, doctor.'

'Right, you are to stay there. I'll come straight out.'

'Very good, doctor,' she answered quite meekly. 'Goodbye.'

I rang through to Fred. 'Miss Spencer's had an accident on Brendon Hill. She says she's all right but I've said I'll get out there. Can you cope? There are about a dozen in the waiting-room. I'll ring Charles's home and see if they can pick him up on his rounds, to come to help.'

'OK Andy, of course you must go and see how she is. I'll manage. Will you just tell them to come in when I ring?'

There were fewer cars then than now and 'speed-cops' were a rarity. Just as well, I thought, as I roared through the downland lanes to Brendon Hill. I only had one near miss and that was a stray cow. As I rounded the bend at the bottom, I was horrified to see Miss Spencer's little Morris half-way up the hill on the wrong side of the road, with the roof flattened and the windscreen out.

I pulled up at the garden gate of the cottage opposite and ran up the path to the door. An elderly man opened it and I could see Miss Spencer inside, sitting by the fire burning in an old open grate, drinking from a cup.

Her clothes were disarrayed. Her usually neat, grey hair was untidy, with the coil at the back of her head undone and dangling loosely down her back. Somehow this shocked me more than if she'd broken an arm. Her spectacles were bent but unbroken. She smiled at me rather wanly.

'How kind of you, doctor, to come so quickly.' Then, with more vigour 'Now cheer up. I haven't broken anything.'

'What happened?' I demanded. The old countryman was pouring another cup of tea. He handed it to me.

'I seed it all master. Lady were coming down hill all nice and steady and this 'ere van come roarin' up; 'e took corner well over on 'er side tryin' to pass tractor wot was ahead of 'im, going real slow. Lady 'ad to go up the bank. 'It 'er rear mudguard with 'is front 'e did. 'Fore yer could say Jack Robinson, she were over on 'er top, then, quick as I sez it, back on 'er wheels again an' chargin' over t'other side of road. But next thing, out she gits and walks over to me at gate. Bit staggery-like she were, swimey, but cool, she were cool as a cucumber. "'ave you a telephone please?" she asks. Well, I 'ave cos me son 'ad it put in since me wife died, so I could call 'im if I needed 'im in 'mergency, so we rung you, zur.'

'I must thank you, you have been really kind. But didn't the van stop?'

'No zur, 'e never stopped – went on up the 'ill as if Old Nick were on 'is tail.'

'Did you get his number?'

'No I never – not proper – you see, me eyes ain't what they used to be. But I see it were a green and white van an' I think one letter of the number were "Y".'

I looked anxiously at Miss Spencer. She was very white and was sitting huddled up in the wooden armchair looking into the fire, her half-empty tea-cup on her lap.

'Do you feel able to walk again now, Miss Spencer, or would you like me to get an ambulance?'

'No doctor, of course I can walk.' She rose rather unsteadily and carefully put the cup and saucer on the table.

'Let me hold your arm. I shall take you straight home.' For once, I was in charge and she was going to do what I said. We steered a wobbly course to the door and I turned to the old man.

'Thank you very much indeed for all your help. You must

let me make you a return. Would you tell me your name please?'

'Me name's Wells, Samuel Wells, but I don't want none o' that, zur. If we can't do something for a poor body what's in need, it's a bad day for us all. You take good care of the lady now.'

'Well thank you again, we won't forget your kindness.'

I went in first and broke the news to old Mrs Spencer as the brother was out, and then insisted that her daughter went to bed. We rang her own country doctor, and then I got through to the surgery and gave them the news.

'I'm sure she should stay off for at least a week,' I told Charles.

'I quite agree. You tell her from me that we'll manage – but I don't know how,' he added.

That was a week, the memory of which only time will erase.

The poor lass from the employment agency did her best but she really hadn't a clue. Her typing was first class; she was willing, she was pretty and she was kind but there her qualifications ended.

Ladies of sixty were sent in with maternity record notes; some records disappeared entirely in the hinterlands of the filing system, only to surface months later. Visits were accepted for patients with minor ailments who would have been very happy with a firm word of advice and we spent hours in the town looking for patients with non-existent addresses and knocking at the doors of total strangers. There were several near punch-ups when people got sent in out of turn.

We double-checked all referrals. Our temporary helper had been a typist-telephonist in a department store and her knowledge of medical terminology was nil. The layout was impeccable but the information obscure.

Amid the gloom, one or two of these letters brought a welcome touch of hilarity to our work. Fred and I were reading the latest together in his room. He smiled as he handed me one.

'I'm sure Mr Hempstead would agree that his hernia is abominable, but what I dictated was abdominal.'

I showed him an X-ray request.

'This should give the radiologist a laugh. "Right humorous. ?Fracture of neck." '

'What about this?' said Fred. 'I thought the postman's chest pain was probably pleurodynia but I suppose Miss Smallweed's version could be right. She's got "plural dinner"!'

The last one for correction really hit the jackpot. I remembered Mr Johnson. He was a small, inoffensive clerk who suffered from attacks of palpitation; he also had a large and loud-voiced wife. Miss Smallweed's diagnosis was probably more accurate than mine. I suggested to the cardiologist that he had 'auricular fibrillation' but her shorthand recorded his trouble as 'auricular tribulation'.

Three pale, exhausted wrecks waited for news of Miss Spencer's recovery. On Saturday, her doctor rang us to say that he thought she could come back on Monday. Charles is not a demonstrative man, but Miss Spencer found a huge bunch of roses waiting for her when she arrived at 8.30 on Monday morning.

Sadly, her insurance was only third party and her little old Morris was a write-off. We couldn't trace the van that hit her. She insisted she could come in by bus, but Charles paid for her to come by taxi in the morning and one of us took her back after the evening surgery.

I don't know how long this would have been kept up if Charles hadn't gone to Tanbury market to buy some ducklings. He had a pond at the back of his garden, where he kept ducks as he liked the eggs. I think he also liked watching the birds sculling in the pond. It brought back memories.

He told us what happened next day in his usual laconic style.

'I was going round the market and I'd decided on some muscovies, when I saw "It", down a side street where the traders park their vans. Green and white stripes and the number JDY 605. I went quietly round and had a look. There was a dent on the offside wing, and it had been repainted. I was just peering at it when I heard a voice behind me.

' "What d'you think you're doin', mate?" He was a big bloke with side-whiskers, in a flashy suit, standing looking at me from about a yard away.

'I said, "Can you kindly tell me where your van was at eight o'clock on Monday morning two weeks ago?"

' "I don't 'ave to answer your b—— questions. You can b—— well push off." And he took me by the lapels of my jacket and stuck his face unpleasantly close and began forcing me backwards.

'I remembered a little judo trick from my undergraduate days. I thought I'd try it. I grabbed his wrists and dropped backward helping him on his way over my head with my right foot. He landed on his back; fortunately for him there was a pile of old cardboard boxes to break his fall so he wasn't hurt – much. But he was absolutely winded.

'I walked off pretty smartish and got round to the police station and told them about the van. The sergeant at the desk called a couple of constables and we went back to the market.

'Now, this is the best bit. The thug who went for me, he and his mate, were packing up their stall like mad in a rush to get away, but when the policemen arrived and looked at the van, they found a load of electrical gadgets inside under a tarpaulin. They recognized it as stuff taken from a van stolen near Maidstone, the day before Miss Spencer's accident.

'They arrested the two men and I think they've discovered where they've stashed the rest of the haul. The police said something about a reward offered by the insurance company for information leading to the arrest of the thieves and re-covery of the stolen goods.'

A month later, Charles got a letter of thanks from the General Accident Fire and Theft and a cheque for £400. After a struggle, Miss Spencer accepted it as a contribution towards a new (second-hand) Morris to replace the old one. The old countryman in the cottage on Brendon Hill is no doubt still wondering who sent him a ton of coal for his open fire.

It took a lot more persuasion to get Miss Spencer to accept an assistant in the office.

'But I really don't need any help, Dr Semple,' she said.

'I know you don't, but *we* will if you take it into your head to get involved in another robbery.' Charles was on form. 'We can't do without you, but if you train an understudy it will be better than nothing.'

Miss Spencer at last admitted that she did know of a Mrs Badger who was a trained secretary, whose family had grown up and who was looking for some part-time work, so we engaged her. Her typing was excellent, she did shorthand as well. She was always cheerful but, when she was in charge alone on the day we persuaded Miss Spencer to take off each week, the peace and tranquillity of the surgery was shattered.

It was just like the effect of a stranger in Charles's duck-run: everything went up in the air. Not that Mrs Badger minded. She loved it. She was at her best with people standing waiting, the telephone going, and the doctors buzzing for patients. For her it was a trial of strength, a test of stamina. But for us – as Charles said, 'I think I'll take a bottle of Mist. Spenceri – I need it!'

8
Situations Vacant: Plumbing Engineer required

'Some days are sent to try us', says Mrs Clout, who is our home help. Brought up in the Salvation Army, she has a robust approach to life, and she needs it.

As a child she must have suffered a spinal injury, as she has a marked kyphosis shortening her by several inches. Her daughter was a polio victim and has deformed leg muscles.

Her husband is a van-driver and his wages have never topped £6 a week. Mrs Clout knows all about trying days.

Early on in the morning I knew this was going to be one of those days, so far as I was concerned.

'Please have a look at the cistern in the downstairs loo before you go – it's leaking,' Elisabeth said to me at breakfast.

'OK love,' I mumbled through toast and marmalade. Finishing my coffee en route, I went to have a look. The supply-pipe was dripping at its connection. I got a spanner from the car boot and gave the nut a good wrench to tighten the joint. That tug twisted off the corroded pipe and a deluge of rusty brown water poured down on my upturned face.

'Quick, lend me a hand!' I yelled, trying vainly to stem the flow with a handkerchief. Mrs Clout, who'd come early to spring-clean, got there first, with Elisabeth close behind, and the heartless pair just stood there, convulsed with mirth at my dripping Red Indian countenance.

'Go and turn off the water,' I begged, and Mrs Clout dived into the cupboard under the stairs and turned off the stop-cock. What a mess! Rusty water staining the walls and lying in pools on the floor. I couldn't stay to help swab it up – I had to wash, do a quick change and get off to the surgery to collect my visits for the day.

It was a usual round: chest complaints, sore throats, gastro-enteritis. I was in one house writing a prescription for a chap with lumbago when the telephone rang in the hall.

'Doctor, it's for you.'

It was Miss Spencer.

'Could you go at once to Mrs Gould at 15 West Park Avenue? A neighbour called in and found her collapsed.'

The neighbour opened the door. 'Oh poor Mrs Gould, I didn't know what to do.' She blushed. 'She's in the smallest room and I can't move her, but I've given her a pillow.'

The door was ajar and there was Mrs Gould lying sideways jammed between the wall and the pan. Her nose seemed to be smelling a rose in the printed wallpaper. She was very brave.

'Have you hurt yourself badly, Mrs Gould? Do you feel you have broken anything?'

'No doctor, but I think I have had a slight stroke. My left arm and leg went sort of helpless and I fell off the seat.'

She must have weighed fifteen stones. I felt so sorry seeing her like this, that I tried to do the heroic he-man stuff and get her out single-handed. I should have waited for the ambulance men.

'Put your good arm round my neck,' I told her.

I got astride the seat and bent over. With one great heave up she came, but as I did it, I felt as if a dagger had been stuck in my lumbar region. I gasped for a moment and then the pain subsided so I carried her out and dumped her on the bed. We arranged for help and then I went back to the car. As I put my foot on the accelerator I found I couldn't feel it. At the same time, a red-hot poker began to bore its way down the back of my thigh, through the calf and out at my big toe. I got home somehow and limped up the steps.

That afternoon our orthopaedic consultant came round. I ruefully told him my tale.

'There's one born every minute.' He looked at me cheerfully when he'd finished his examination. 'A disc – probably between lumbar four and five. Bed for you, and analgesics.' He gave me some pethidine tablets.

That night as I lay with the burning pain only a little dulled, trying not to disturb Elisabeth, I thought over the strange fact that loos seemed to have dogged my life, so to speak.

I got myself locked in one as a child and was nearly concussed when my dad broke down the door to let me out. I remembered the Christmas party when we were teenagers. The game was sardines and my highly original hiding-place on the scullery roof ridge had to be reached through the loo window. I couldn't get back when the window jammed. My mother had something to say when she saw the state of my rain-sodden best suit.

In spite of the pain in my leg I chuckled quietly to myself when I thought of that Corps Camp on Salisbury Plain many years before, and the joker who waited in the top cubicle until the automatic flush sluiced under the line of seats. Then he lit a newspaper and sent it down the channel and listened to the shouts and yells of the unlucky occupants of the other cubicles. Incidentally, I was not that joker.

My mind wandered off to Africa – yes, even there, in that far-off place, I could not avoid the hoodoo of the loo.

There, they were well-constructed little huts placed in secluded but often charming spots down the garden, but they concealed fearsome pits beneath, thirty to forty feet deep.

Elisabeth had had a narrow escape. Toilet rolls were expensive and only to be bought forty-five miles away in the township. A pile of magazines were in the loo in lieu, as one might say. She had entered the little hut, moved the magazines and immediately flung herself outside with a scream. A small black mamba lay coiled among the papers. Our imperturbable woodcutter nonchalantly despatched the intruder with the blunt end of his axe and dropped him into the depths.

The memory of this incident was still fresh in my mind when a week later I was seated in the same hut. Without warning and quite involuntarily I broke the All Africa record for the sitting jump, letting out a wild whoop of fear. I had suddenly felt a sharp jab in the region of my gluteus maximus. To my intense relief – for I had visions of a mamba bite – I saw there was a little round hole in the woodwork, and protruding from it were the large pincers of a white ant. He had obviously objected to the sudden cutting-off of his light and air and had nipped me in retaliation.

We had to cut away all the wooden seat and reconstruct a new one and this was just as well. What might have happened if the white ants had further weakened it is too awful to contemplate.

But this did not end my saga.

Shortly afterwards, we were staying on a Kenya farm with some friends, Helen and Henry, for a short holiday. They had a wireless and we appreciated even the overseas news when we'd not heard it for some years.

The aerial was slung from a high podocarpus tree to a pole

near the house. We were finishing our tea in the lounge when the sky went dark and a tropical storm burst on us. Unwisely, I chose that very moment to pop out to the loo.

There was a blinding flash as the thunder exploded overhead. Immediately after there was another crash inside the house. The others didn't know what had happened, but I did. I was still in the loo. The lightning had struck the aerial, jumped to a metal pipe leading into the loo and shattered the porcelain pan to smithereens. Fortunately for me, I was not in situ at that precise moment.

Henry came back later with us to the mission. He had pretensions to being a water-diviner and we badly needed water. Rain-water tanks were running out and we had resorted to donkeys to bring it up from the river in petrol tins. We were cock-a-hoop when he divined water just near the hospital.

We weren't worried when we reached forty feet in the digging. The loos on the station were as deep as that and they held no water. The hardy workmen went on down. They had no boarding to shore up the walls, they just cut steps as they went down. One man on top hauled the soil up in a bucket, and emptied it. I went down myself and the claustrophobic sensation of looking up at the patch of sky overhead with the stars showing faintly in the daytime was quite frightening.

Still they dug on – sixty feet, seventy – but, unlike Isaac's well-diggers in the book of Genesis, they found no water. We gave up at eighty feet. Rather than waste a perfectly good hole, we decided to put it to another use, and now we feel we can claim a place in the *Guinness Book of Records* for the deepest pit loo in the world.

However, the Africa loo view was not entirely dark. Before we left Kenya almost my last effort to improve things on the station was to install two chromium-plated 'flush johns'. We bought them in Nairobi for a song. They had been part of a huge consignment flown out in US transport planes to meet the needs of their desert troops in North Africa. It was a pity they didn't find out first that there was no running water in the desert. However, by then we had developed running water from a primitive but highly efficient pumping system which raised water seven hundred feet from our river, and the loos worked a treat.

I drifted off into slumber . . .

To my intense relief, when I awoke, the pain in my leg was nearly gone. The prolapsed disc had somehow moved in the night and the pressure was off the roots of my sciatic nerve.

But, sad to say, I have never recovered the friskiness and feeling in my big toe and I have been unable to turn on the hot tap in the bath with it ever since.

However, I intend to avoid lifting people out of loos in future.

We got Mrs Gould some special chromium-plated wall handles for her loo as well, and there is now little danger of her falling off again. I was glad when she got a good deal of use back in her arm and leg, and a niece to come and share her home to look after her. It was an added safeguard.

9

He got his medal
in the end

It was one of those typically English days of seeping rain in early November; the last few leaves were drifting down on the garden of the old house standing a quarter of a mile from the front. They lay unswept and sodden on the path to the front door. I trod through them to the steps, cracked and sunk to uneven surfaces by the subsidence of years.

I scanned the little name-plates and found 'Jenkins – 4' at the top. I pressed the bell. It was too far away for me to hear it ring, so I pushed open the front door and started up the stairs.

Each flight was different. Up to the first floor the treads had a covering of clean, well-polished lino – I pictured the residents as perhaps a prim retired clerk and his wife. Next I was walking on a rather florid carpet, good quality but needing a brush – who lived there? It suggested a flouncy, middle-aged shop assistant. Then it was boards and tatty lino littered with cigarette-ends – perhaps a couple of students? The last flight had a threadbare carpet, drab but clean, and I got the feeling that here was an old couple, tired but hanging on to frayed gentility.

There was a little brass knocker on the door. The bell must have worked because the door opened as soon as I knocked.

'Mrs Jenkins?'

'You must be the new doctor,' she said. 'Please come in' and then, *sotto voce*, 'Would you mind coming in here first?' She led me into the kitchen.

'Doctor, my husband hasn't seen anyone for years about his health. Doesn't take to doctors, in fact, doesn't get on with anybody very well,' she said apologetically. 'And he has a bit of a temper. He's not been himself lately and there's a nasty lump under his ear which worries me. I couldn't get him to the surgery so I hope you don't mind me calling you.'

'That's all right, Mrs Jenkins.'

I braced myself for a not-too-pleasant interview. According to his record-card Mr Jenkins was sixty-nine. His last visit to a doctor had been twenty years ago in Bradford.

'We had a small business up in Bradford,' Mrs Jenkins explained. 'We hadn't many friends there so when Albert retired we thought we'd come south to Wilverton. It was the one place we liked when we had our holidays. We didn't have very many,' she added pathetically.

A rough voice called, 'Milly! Who's that you're talking to?'

'I'd better go and see him, Mrs Jenkins,' I whispered.

I knocked on the bedroom door and walked in. He was a big, heavy-jowled man. I said, 'I'm Doctor Hamilton, Mr Jenkins – come to have a look at you.'

He stuck out his jaw. 'You won't find much wrong wi' me,' he growled. 'It were Milly, she would send for you.'

He was sitting up in bed with a dressing-gown over his

pyjamas. One or two old account books lay on the table by his bedside. It looked as if he had been going over old business from his Bradford shop days.

'Well, now I'm here I'd better examine you.'

From the end of the bed I could see that the angle of his right jaw was filled in with a swelling and my heart sank. I started with his chest and heart as he reluctantly opened his pyjama jacket for me to examine him. His heart was in good shape, but his chest was noisy and he coughed when I asked him to take a deep breath. By the books on the table lay an old pipe with matches and a pouch, and the room smelt of stale tobacco smoke.

'May I have a look at your mouth now?'

He opened it, and behind his yellowed teeth my torch picked out a nasty whitish ulcer on the right side of his tongue.

'Do you mind if I put a finger in your mouth? It's quite clean.'

I felt his tongue. The ulcer was hard and irregular. He winced and I pulled out my finger.

'Hurts a bit, that does,' he said.

Lastly I felt his neck under his chin; there was a hard mass in the angle of the jaw and lumps of glands farther down his neck as well.

'How much do you smoke, Mr Jenkins?'

'Well, not much.'

'Well, how much?'

'Not more than four or five ounces a week, but Ah've been doing that for donkey's years – never done me any harm.'

'Well, you've got bronchitis you know,' I was playing myself in. 'And you've also got a nasty ulcer on your tongue and it's affected the glands in your neck. I'd like you to see a specialist about it.'

He'd got advanced cancer of the tongue and the glands in his neck were invaded. He would have to have most of the tongue removed and radiation to the glands, but even then his chances were small. He might not survive an operation with that chest of his.

'Now then, doctor. Ah want it straight – what's the matter with me?'

I don't tell patients lies, but there are ways of gradually introducing the truth so that they don't have to take it all at once. But this was a man who seemed to have been fighting odds all his life; he wanted it outright with no flannel.

'Mr Jenkins, I am afraid you've got a growth on your tongue. It has spread to your neck glands and it must be dealt with urgently.'

He blinked. Then he said much more quietly, 'What are my chances?'

'Well, they're not good, but you could be all right for a time. It's a serious operation and you would have to lose most of your tongue.'

'Right then doctor, that settles it.' He took a deep breath. 'No operation for me. Ah'll just bide at home. Milly's a good wife although ah've given her a bit of a life. She'll care for me.'

Milly was standing just outside the half-open door and at that she came in.

'"Course I will, Albert, but you take doctor's advice now.'

'Don't you worry, woman,' he said roughly, but kindly 'Ah knows what Ah'm doin'.'

'Well, if you won't change your mind, Mr Jenkins, I'll have to leave it at that for the moment. I'll come in a week's time and see how you are.'

'Right, doctor,' he said affably, 'you do that, and . . thanks, you're straight you are.'

There wasn't much change when I saw him the following week, but he was thinner and he winced when I touched that swollen neck. I didn't hurry off but stopped to listen to his complaints. He seemed to be responding to friendship, and his anger and resentment slowly subsided. We found a common interest in rugby football as he'd been an ardent supporter of the Northern League until he came to live in West Sussex.

'Reckon our Bradford boys'd see off some of you namby-pamby clubs if they 'ad their chance.'

He was spoiling for a good fight.

'Go on, they aren't all that tough – look at the rests they get when the game's stopped for the tackles.' I wasn't going to let him have it all his own way. 'Besides *we* do it for fun, your blokes are paid!'

He looked for a moment as if he was going to blow a gasket. Then he grinned: ' 'Aven't enjoyed meself like this for long enough.'

He began to go downhill rapidly, and as the sensory nerves got involved in the growth his pain increased. At first he wouldn't have any pain-relieving drugs, but after a while he consented to have aspirin and codeine and this helped for a bit.

Milly fussed about, doing everything for him and one day he said to me, 'Ah've seen she's all right, doctor. Ah've a bit put by. She's no cause to worry. She's a good girl. Pity we had no time to have kids. They'd be a comfort to her now.'

I had begun to visit every other day and I could see he was losing his iron control. On one visit, just before I left, I said:

'Mr Jenkins, would you be offended if we said a prayer together? It might help.'

'Well, doctor, do if you like.' He was gruff, but he put his hands together and closed his eyes.

I thanked God for his nearness and that, in spite of everything, we could still know that he loved us because he sent his own Son, Jesus, to our world and allowed him to suffer and die on our behalf. I asked God to bring peace to them both, and to free Mr Jenkins from fear and send him relief from pain. I wondered what his reaction would be as he had never signified that he gave a thought to God.

It was a short stumbling prayer. At the end he said 'Amen' quite heartily.

On the next visit, as I was closing my bag, Mr Jenkins said, 'What about another prayer then, doc?'

After that it became a regular thing which he looked forward to. In our prayers we spoke of Jesus' compassion, his forgiveness and the welcome we could expect when we turn to him in real trust.

Six weeks went by and Mr Jenkins was getting pretty

71

weak. His stalwart frame was fading away, but his mind was clear in spite of increasing doses of pain-killing drugs. He was needing morphia and the doses got steadily bigger.

One day he turned to me.

'Ah'm going to tell you something, doctor – something Ah've never told a soul before. When Ah was a boy, Ah was a raight religious lad. Sang in t'choir and went to Sunday school.

'One day vicar said to us, "Now you boys, I want you to help collect money for a mission in Nigeria. The boy that gets the most will be given a medal."

'Ah worked raight hard to collect money – doing errands, chopping firewood, anything that I could do for a penny or two, and when they counted up the money, Ah'd won. But, do you know, Ah never got my medal – never. Ah left the Sunday school and Ah've hated church ever since.

'Can Ah tell you what you coming and talking and praying has meant? It's as if Ah've lived all my life in a sort of darkness and now the light's come back. Ah don't mind dying now.'

He smiled his twisted smile and for a moment his face looked quite radiant.

'Perhaps Ah'll get my medal on t'other side.'

It wasn't long for him after that. He slipped into a coma one morning and when I went back in the evening he had just gone. I stood with his wife by the bedside. Her eyes were filled with tears as she looked up at me and silently squeezed my hand.

I walked away through the sodden leaves to the gate. What a small wrong had darkened this man's life and what a small candle had dispelled the darkness at the last.

10
Algernon

When we arrived at Wilverton and after we had drawn breath, we looked around for a church to go to.

I was visiting near the front when I passed a nondescript building, which looked like a furniture repository. I stopped for a moment as it struck me as oddly out of place among the hotels and boarding-houses. Over the door I could read 'Public Swimming-Bath 1903'. At the side, a flaking block of stone bore the inscription 'Laid by Mr Anthony Bunkin, Mayor of Wilverton' and in small print, barely readable, 'Larcumbe and Weevil Builders'. There was a small blue board screwed to the door. 'Wilverton Temporary Church', it said.

It was only a quarter of a mile from our flat so it looked a likely berth for us. Charles and Fred had churches of their own up at the other end of the town but Fred said the Wilverton vicar was a live wire. I said, rather feebly, 'Dangerous, in a swimming-bath!' However, we thought we'd have a go.

Next Sunday, there we were, all sitting quietly near the back – that is, all except Barney, who was under the seat speculatively inspecting the shoe-laces of the person in the pew behind with evil intent. I wasn't anticipating it when a hand fell on my shoulder. I half-expected a whispered message to go and see a patient, but a large beaming face was close to mine and it said, 'Glad to meet you. May I have your name and address?'

This was our first contact with the Reverend Algernon Greenfield, but it certainly wasn't the last. The very next week he was round to visit us. He was a tall, powerfully-built man with a battered face and ruddy complexion. He looked a typical old rugger player – and indeed, that's just what he was.

Charles informed me that in the dim and distant past,

Algernon had got up a team of parsons to play a team of doctors. I gather there was a serious rending of the cloth by the ferocious medics.

You didn't get to know Algernon, you felt he was an old friend from the moment he loomed in sight. He was the genuine, original, purpose-built eccentric, quite incapable of doing anything in the orthodox manner.

When the Luftwaffe destroyed his church, it was he who conceived the idea of worshipping in a swimming-bath. Being poised for Matins and Evensong over a tiled abyss must have worried several of the elderly in the congregation, but not Algernon.

He won the children's hearts and their attention early on. He was illustrating the armour of the Christian in his fight against evil. He suddenly bent down in the pulpit and reappeared with an enormous helmet on his head; next he brandished a six-foot sword over the heads of the cowering choir. This knightly impedimenta had been the property of a famous Sussex giant. Algernon had borrowed them from the museum for the occasion.

For all his one-off unpredictability, he was as shrewd as they come. He could see through cant and self-pity like a modern body-scanner and he got away with murder in his candid counsels.

A patient of ours, Edwin Tindall, had lost his wife with a stroke two years before I joined the practice. He had retired early and was living a comfortable life looked after by a competent housekeeper and supported by many friends. These last were getting thinner on the ground because of his habit of expatiating on his deceased wife's virtues and bemoaning her loss on every possible occasion.

Only Algie could have done it. He stopped Tindall one day when he was in full spate: 'Edwin my boy,' (they were roughly the same age), 'you really must stop going over the past. Elsie is safe and happy and you're simply refusing to accept God's plan for you. You're like someone going round being sick over people, and they don't like it!' Now if *I'd* done that . . .

It remains a fact that from that day Edwin changed his

tune, and instead of being a querulous bore he started being useful and a pleasure to meet. The last time I saw him, he was arm in arm with two old men from the blind home, and they were all marching along the front laughing their heads off.

Charles inveigled me into helping him with a Christian boys' club. It seemed obvious that Algie must be asked to talk to them. One day he came.

He got up slowly, looking round enquiringly at everyone and then he suddenly said: 'How many bones are there in a giraffe's neck?' Attention was absolutely rivetted. 'Do you know? Don't you know? You don't?' Long pause. 'Well, neither do I.' Fury and frustration in the ranks! 'But I do know something.' Hope rekindled. 'They've got the same number as we have.' Would the boys ever forget the lesson? Tall or short, clever or dim-witted, they were all the same inside.

After this we had the traditional bun-fight and organized games, which is just another way of saying a near-riot. They were determined to get their own back on Algernon for not knowing the number of the giraffe's cervical vertebrae.

'Sir, sir, if we ask you a riddle and you can't answer, will you do a forfeit?'

Algernon, of course, dropped himself right in it. 'OK what's the riddle?'

'What's black and dangerous?'

'Hmm . . . don't know.'

A chorus: 'A crow with a machine-gun. Now you've got to pay the forfeit.'

They stuck two chairs together with their seats touching and announced.

'You see these chairs, sir? Got to take off your shoes and jump over them.'

I don't know whether they thought Algie would back out but he was made of sterner stuff. He whipped off his brightly-polished black brogues, revealing a pair of beautiful purple socks and, nimble as a mountain-goat, he leapt the chairs amid rapturous applause.

'Sir, sir, we caught you. You only had to jump the shoes!' – as if Algernon didn't know!

I attributed his ruddy complexion to his habit of bathing in the sea before breakfast all the year round. He was one of our patients, and when he got a cold followed quickly by pneumonia, I knew the time had come for him to give up this routine.

When he was convalescent, I made a final call. He was sitting at the window which looked out to sea. He had some drawing paper with sketches on beside him on a small table.

'Don't say it.' He held up a finger with a smile. 'I know I'll have to stop the daily dip, but there's something I want to show you. It's my vision for our rebuilt church. We live by the sea, Andrew; this is something we ought to capitalize on. We don't want some static, ghetto-like concept for the building. I dreamt that God was telling us like Peter to launch out – not stay cosily tied up in harbour, and that's what our new church has got to express.'

He wasn't much of a draughtsman, but I could see from his sketches what he had in mind: the superstructure of a great ship! Maybe it doesn't sound very feasible, but when the architect's preliminary drawings were presented, they really did convey the impression of the upper parts of a majestic liner.

But Algernon's vision was still a long way from realization in stone and brick. Government war-damage compensation went nowhere near to paying for the style of building that had been conceived. Funds came in very slowly, despite Algernon's unsurpassed ability to get people to give.

It was positively dangerous to let him know of a need. I made the cardinal error of mentioning to him one day that our furniture supply for the home we hoped to have one day was practically nil. The response of the congregation to his appeal for a young ex-missionary's family furnishings would have equipped *three* reasonably-sized houses.

But his own response to need wasn't always to ask; very often it was to act. The Misses Beckwith were a case in point.

They were two elderly maiden ladies sharing a very small flat. They were not parishioners of Algernon's but that didn't worry him. Miss Celia Beckwith spent every day and most nights looking after her sister who was in the late stages of an inoperable breast cancer. She could not now get out of bed unaided even to use the commode. Celia wouldn't allow her sister to go to hospital and they couldn't afford private nursing. Consequently, the good woman was being worn to a shred. She never got a break.

At eight o'clock one evening, a knock came on the door of their flat. She opened it cautiously on the chain; there stood Algernon. He had a dressing-gown over his arm and a pair of carpet slippers in his hand.

'May I come in?'

'Oh yes, do come in, Mr Greenfield.'

Miss Celia was quite overcome and, slipping the chain off, she stood aside. But Algernon did not walk through into the lounge. With his free hand he gently took Miss Celia's arm.

'There, my dear, you are going to bed and your sister will be looked after so you have nothing to worry about.'

'But, but who – ?'

'Now, now. She will be properly cared for. I was attached to an emergency dressing station in the first World War and I understand nursing.'

Still protesting feebly, I gather, Miss Celia allowed herself to be sent to bed. Algernon did his stuff, commode and all, taking forty winks in an armchair between chores. A still-bewildered Celia gave me the full story next morning when I was checking her sister's condition.

He loved to make fun at his own expense, and called himself 'the Prince of Beggars'. Yet the ironical thing was that the church's greatest need was met without Algernon saying a word about it.

The ambulance men called me one afternoon in the spring because they felt doubtful about the state of a man's hip. He was a visitor on a two-week holiday in Wilverton, and he'd slipped while walking along the front. In fact, when I pressed his pelvis, I felt that he had undoubtedly cracked a pubic ramus. X-ray confirmed this, and it was really a matter of his lying and sitting around in his holiday flatlet with his wife to help him until the bone healed sufficiently for him to go home to Birmingham. He was bored and frustrated and his holiday was spoilt.

Hearing about him, Algernon brought a breath of fresh air and companionship into his room by friendly visits. He discovered that the man had been a clothing retailer who had done very well in business before retiring and selling out, as there were no children to carry on the business.

A year later, Algernon received a letter from a firm of solicitors. His visitor friend had died and the church had been left £60,000 in his will, and another £60,000 to come which was still in trust to his wife during her lifetime. With the war-damage payment, it was now possible to 'lay down the keel' of the new Wilverton church.

'And I never asked the dear fellow for a penny,' said Algernon.

11
Easter

Up from the grave He arose,
With a mighty triumph o'er His foes;
He arose a Victor from the dark domain,
And He lives for ever with His saints to reign!
He arose! He arose!
Hallelujah! Christ arose!

We pulled out all the stops for that last chorus. Peter, Sarah and even little Barney, as far as he was able, were all joining in.

I enjoy my singing, even though my neighbours in church seem less enthusiastic. Towards the end of the third verse I got a nudge from Elisabeth. She nodded towards the small man in the pew in front. I glanced down. His head was hunched forward into his shoulders like a seaman bending before the blast. I took the hint and dropped the volume a few decibels.

We left the church at the end of the service and went out into the spring sunshine. It was Easter Day and the theme of the sermon had been simple: 'If Jesus Christ is not alive, I'm wasting my time preaching and you're wasting yours listening. Go home and dig the garden, have a good time while you can, because when you're dead, you're dead. But if he is risen and you believe it, your life will never be the same again.' It was typical Algernon stuff – straight talking and no padding.

We wandered thoughtfully towards the beach. The tide was out and a huge expanse of sand stretched far beyond the shingle to the greeny-blue line of the sea. Barney began contentedly to make sand-pies on the dry patch near the shingle. Sarah wandered off collecting little pink shells, while Peter edged slowly towards a huge concourse of seabirds standing three hundred yards along the shore. There would be greater and lesser black backs, herring, common and black-headed gulls, several kinds of tern, red-billed oyster-catchers and dappled turnstones, but he wanted to see how many waders he could spot as well, before the outlying ones took fright and led a swirling cloud into the air to land farther down the beach.

It was peaceful, and despite the north-easterly breeze, the sun made it warm enough for Elisabeth and me to sit comfortably on the stones. I didn't want to get my only decent pair of suede shoes stained with sea-water, so I just lay back with my hands behind my head and relaxed.

Memories of other Easters drifted through my mind.

I was a twelve-year-old again and the three of us – John, Graham and me (Rat, Grimey and Tub) – were biking into the country. It was Easter Monday and we rode off into the woods on the hillside above the Eynsford Valley in Kent. We'd got a picnic which included raw sausages ready for impaling on sticks and blackening over a little camp-fire. My knowledge of Christianity was minimal but, as it was Easter, after our lunch, I carved a little cross on a sapling with my sheath knife and added my initials underneath. I didn't really know why.

My mind leapt the years to the late 1930s. I was walking with my unruly crew in the strangest garb up the little Broadland hill to Ranworth Church, famous for its priceless illuminated missal, each page inscribed by the monks on a single sheepskin. We officers were a group of undergraduates running a cruise for boys, teaching them to sail and sharing the secrets of the Christian life.

I sat in the church trying to catch a glimpse of my girl-friend, Elisabeth. I could just see the top of her fair hair amongst the other girls on the other side of the nave. She was vice-commodore of a girls' cruise. We were all sharing Sunday morning service.

We all stood up as, down the aisle, came the choir followed by the old vicar and behind him a truly magnificent figure. It was Jack Collins, former rowing blue, six foot eight in height. An immense white surplice draped his giant form, shining in the sunlight from the windows and tactfully covering his sweater and blue sailing trousers, as he strode to his seat in the chancel.

Again my mind switched . . . The years had gone by and I was once again in church, only this time, it was a building made of mud and sticks with a tin roof which grew unbearably hot under the African sun. My good friend Job, the gap-toothed, pock-marked, jovial soul, was holding a hundred men, women and children spellbound with his brilliant, witty sermon. He was a natural. He could preach at the drop of a hat, but it came out of a heart full of devotion to God.

As I listened to him I felt a hand pulling my sleeve. I swivelled round on the log seat. There was my hospital orderly, Isaiah, beckoning me. I followed him quietly outside.

'Bwana, they have brought in a girl, *imione mising*. She is very sick. I couldn't wait till the end of the service.'

'All right Isaiah, where is she?'

'In the examination-room, Dokitare.'

I found a girl of about fourteen, dressed in a rawhide skirt and cape, lying in a delirium on the examination-room table.

'*Kigomian betusiek ata*? How many days has she been ill?' I asked the father, who had brought her with the help of relatives on a makeshift stretcher of poles and skins from a section of the tribe about thirty miles away. He held up his hand with the thumb tucked between the first two fingers.

'Five days! Why did you not bring her before?'

Isaiah spoke quietly.

'They have been trying the *jepkerijot* – the medicine woman – first.'

At that moment the child's body stiffened and her back arched like a bow, her teeth bared in a ghastly grin and her breathing became mere shallow grunts, then ceased altogether for about half a minute.

'She's got tetanus, Isaiah.'

We pulled aside her skin robe and there was a horrible sore on her thigh, covered with the usual dressing of cowdung.

I had never seen a case of tetanus before. In England, it is a rare disease. We had no antitoxin and it would have been of doubtful value if we had had some. The poor girl's body relaxed and she began to breathe again at last.

I quickly gave her an injection of morphia, knowing that we must quieten her irritated brain, and stop the spasms if possible. The morphia would be slow to take effect and it would only partially control the horrible contractions.

'Isaiah, fetch the chloroform and anaesthetic mask please.'

It was a losing battle I knew, but I must spare this poor girl all the suffering I could. The father had gone outside and was sitting on the edge of the concrete verandah.

Isaiah and I watched the stricken face intently. The muscles at the corner of her mouth began to twitch again.

I quickly put the mask over her face and began dropping on the chloroform. The sickly-sweet smell filled the sunlit room. The twitching slowed and then it began to increase again and she went into another ghastly spasm. She was taking no breaths so the chloroform was not being inhaled.

I took off the mask and waited. At last she relaxed on the couch again and her breathing jerkily restarted.

We fought on but we lost. A few spasms later, she collapsed once more but she did not breathe again. I listened to her chest: there was no heartbeat.

We went out to her father, sad, sweating and beaten. Isaiah laid a kindly hand on his shoulder.

'*A-bonyu, kagome lakwa*. My father, the child has died.'

We weren't ready for his response.

He turned fiercely to me.

'You have killed her, white man, you have killed her. I demand compensation!'

Isaiah stiffened. 'Bwana Dokitare has fought to save your child's life and can you speak to him like this?'

'Let me see her,' he answered sullenly.

He went in, stared at the dead girl for a moment, then pulled the skins away from her body to see if we had injured her in any way.

'What is that stink?' he asked Isaiah.

Isaiah showed him the bottle.

'It is the medicine to stop the spasms, old man.'

'Well, she is dead,' he said abruptly and, to my amazement, he roughly undid her necklace and pulled off the steel wire armlets from his daughter's body, wrapped them in his body-cloth and left the room without another word.

'Bwana, he should not go like that,' Isaiah protested. 'He should help bury the body. It is proper, it is the custom.'

'Let him go, Isaiah, he has lost his child. We will bury her.'

Faintly down the breeze came the singing of the last hymn from the church:

'*Kigong'et! Kigong'et! Alleluya, Kigong'et*! He arose! He arose! Hallelujah! Christ arose!'

We looked at each other. We were thinking of the anger and despair of the poor tribesman who did not know the hope those words could bring. . .

'Andy, quick!' Elisabeth was on her feet. I sat up with a jerk. I could see Sarah 200 yards away near some rocks, and against the wind I caught her cry.

'Mummy, Daddy, help me!'

Then I was tearing over the shingle. Near the edge where the tide had reached that morning lay an old frayed length of rope fallen overboard from some ship. It was smeared with black oil but it might be life-saving. I grabbed it as I ran.

Sarah was in a quicksand, and with her struggling she had already sunk above her knees.

'Daddy, Daddy, help me! I'm sinking,' she screamed.

'Darling, stay absolutely still. Now try and fall over backwards.'

She did just as she was told. Ten feet away the sand was still firm.

'Catch!' I hurled the old rope over my head and it fell two feet from her right side. 'Grab it, my darling. Now, can you tie it around you and under your arms?'

She did it very well.

'Now pull the knot round to your back and hold on.'

I dug my heels into the sand behind a rock. I pulled as hard as I could. Elisabeth was with me now. She held on to the shoulders of my jacket and slowly, so slowly, we dragged Sarah out. Her feet and legs came out with a sucking noise, covered with a foul black ooze.

We pulled her gently over the sand and held her tight, while she sobbed out her fear. At last she had recovered. Peter helped her to wash off the black mud in a rock pool. One of her sandals had been left behind in the mud, but what did we care? She was safe.

As we trudged up the beach we saw the notice for the first time: 'Warning, dangerous patches of soft sand. Keep clear.'

Chocolate Easter eggs and hot cross buns for tea helped to dispel the terror of the morning.

When the children were all in their pyjamas that night, we sat on the rug in front of the electric fire and read the first three verses of Psalm 40 together:

'I waited patiently for the Lord;
he turned to me and heard my cry.
He lifted me out of the slimy pit,
out of the mud and mire;

he set my feet on a rock
and gave me a firm place to stand.
He put a new song in my mouth,
a hymn of praise to our God.
Many will see and fear
and put their trust in the Lord.'
It was a sermon and an illustration worthy of Algernon.

12

The Jolly scene

'Doctor Hamilton? This is station control. Sorry for disturbing you, sir. One of our constables has just phoned in. He says he has a man up a tree in Downs Road. Reckons he's had a few. Name of Jolly. Says he's a patient of yours – says it loud and clear, doctor, disturbing the neighbourhood. Constable wants to know, would you come and get him down?'

I swallowed and licked my lips; the watch on the bedside table said 12.25.

'Officer, my climbing days are over. Tell the constable it's the fire brigade he needs, not a doctor.' I caught a snigger on the other end of the line.

'As you say sir, must say I agree. New on the beat, this chap. Will cope. My apologies. Good night.'

I switched out the light and sighed as I lay back on the pillows. Should I have gone? Perhaps I could have talked Frank Jolly down. He wasn't a bad chap when he wasn't hitting the bottle. Oh well – I began to drift off . . . but it wasn't restful sleep. If it was what the psychologists call 'rapid-eye-movement sleep', it was pretty rapid in my case I'd say.

'Brr-Brr.' Oh no!

I grabbed the phone and put the light on again. One o'clock on the dot.

'Yes? Dr Hamilton here.'

'Doctor, sorry to bother you again.' The police officer was positively cringing. 'I've got the fire chief on the blower. He says they've got the man down with an extension ladder but he's fighting drunk. Will you come and give him an injection to quieten him?'

My repentant feeling vanished.

'Officer, tell the fire chief from me that if the combined police and fire services can't control one man – and Jolly isn't all that tough – then I'm not coming to give him an illegal injection to help them. Anyway I should be guilty of an assault on the person. OK?'

'Doctor, my humble apologies. I will give the fire chief your message. Good night.'

It was no good. I quietly got up and went into the kitchen. While the water was boiling for my cup of tea, I sat by the table with my head in my hands. Oh dear, what have I done now? Suppose my home catches fire, will they refuse to come? That bobby: he'll be watching out for me – parking tickets, breaking the speed limit, the lot. One is not very logical at 1.15 a.m.

Frank Jolly was duly done for being drunk and disorderly. My home didn't catch fire, but one week later I was proceeding at a rate of knots to a midder case in the maternity home over on the other side of the town. Curious, how they'd arranged the hospital on one side and the maternity home on the other.

I was buzzing along the top road when I saw the speed-cops' car in my mirror. I dropped from forty to thirty, but my brake-lights must have shown red. The car dogged me for half a mile – right to the home. I pulled up outside and saw with dismay that the police car had halted opposite! I started to walk towards the front door as if in a hurry – which I was. This was persecution! Sheer revenge!

Out of the corner of my eye I saw the window opening by the driver's seat. A large red face looked out.

' 'Ullo, doc. Are you turning out for the old Wilverton team on Saturday, man?'

Those tones could only belong to Sergeant Dai Jones, our burly Welsh forward. I sighed with relief.

'Hullo Dai, nice to see you. Thought you were following me. No, I'm not playing, Dai. I've hung up my boots.'

'Sorry to hear that, doc. See you around.'

In the week that followed I forgot the whole thing. Then Mrs Jolly called me herself one evening. It was only nine o'clock. The pubs weren't closed yet. It must be one of the children in trouble.

'Doctor, would you please come and see Frank?'

'What? Has he had too many again, Mrs Jolly?'

'No, doctor. Please, he's really ill, in pain, bad pain.'

'Right, Mrs Jolly. Just hang on and I'll be round.'

Poor soul. She'd had a life. They had three children, aged ten, nine and eight, and Frank had a good job in a machine tool-makers'. He was actually a very good workman, but he would sail so near the wind and often turn up with a hangover, and I could see that the firm was unlikely to remain tolerant for much longer.

Frank was in bed, flat on his back. There was a strong smell of beer in the room but he wasn't drunk. He was lying dead still; he was pale, and breathing in curious short gasps. His pulse was racing.

'Where's the pain, Frank?'

'All over my tummy, doc,' he jerked out, 'all over.'

I put a hand gently on his umbilical area. He cried out.

His abdominal wall was like a board. I managed to do a rectal examination but it didn't help me. I was sure he'd got a generalized peritonitis – but why so widespread? And why so quickly? He'd been boozing in the pub half an hour before.

'Have you had any indigestion, Frank – in the past, I mean?'

'Nothing much, doctor,' he gasped. 'Just a bit after fish and chips perhaps.'

I couldn't waste any more time with questions.

There was a telephone booth fifty yards down the road, I'd phone from there. I went down the stairs. Mrs Jolly was at the bottom looking up. She was winding her hands in her apron.

'What is it, doctor?'

'Look, Mrs Jolly, Frank's got something nasty in his tummy. He'll have to go to hospital at once, I'm afraid. Probably need an operation. Now don't be upset. He's going to be all right. I'll phone down the road and he'll be in in a jiffy.'

As I opened the door, she collapsed on the bottom step of the stairs and put the back of her hand up to her eyes.

'Oh poor Frank.' Her voice shook with misery and fear.

The house surgeon rang me up at midnight. I'd asked them to tell me what happened.

'You'll never guess what we found in his peritoneal cavity when we opened him up, doctor. Beer – three pints of it. Rather a waste!' Young housemen have a curious sense of humour. 'Perforated ulcer high up on the lesser curvature of the stomach. The chief has done a good job; closed it up, but that's all. He's pretty shocked but the wound's draining well. Not so much beer in the fluid now! Didn't he complain of ulcer symptoms before?'

'No, never. Naturally he was sick a few times after his drinking bouts, but no actual pain. Until I asked him tonight, he'd never mentioned it. He said that fish and chips gave him some pain.'

'Curious . . . Well, he'd better lay off the beer from now on. Nearly had his chips this time. Oops, sorry! Good night.'

Frank survived, and he was home again after a stormy three weeks in hospital. I asked the local Salvation Army Officer to call, and the Army were wonderful organizing help with the children. What was really splendid was that the whole affair really pulled Frank up short. He started going with his wife and the family to the Salvation Army hall and he had a good old-fashioned conversion. He went right off drink and his house began to smarten up and his kiddies lost that hangdog look I was so used to seeing.

Strangely enough though, Mrs Jolly didn't respond. It was her indomitable spirit that had kept the family going in the lean years of Frank's drinking but now she seemed to go flat, withdrawn, as if she had been sucked dry.

It was about nine o'clock again when I got called to their house. This time it was Frank on the phone.

'Doctor, it's not for me this time, thank goodness, but it's the missus. She's acting very strange, sitting on a chair in the kitchen looking at the table. Won't say a word to me. Come and see 'er, doctor, will you?'

'OK. Frank, you keep an eye on her and I'll be with you.'

When Frank opened the front door, I heard a noise in the kitchen and the back door banged. Frank and I ran through and out of the kitchen window we saw Mrs Jolly taking the low fence between their garden and the next like a springbok. I ran back through the house and along the front of the little terrace where they lived. At the end, about ten houses up, I knew there was a lane leading round to the backyards. I' had to use it one day when I couldn't get in by the front door to see a patient.

I charged down the lane just in time to catch Mrs Jolly as she took the last fence. She landed slap on my chest. She didn't struggle, but just burst into tears.

'Don't put me away doctor, don't put me away!'

It was a new situation for me, but I did my best. I patted the back of her head softly and held her up with one arm as her legs were giving way after that remarkable hurdle race.

'No one's going to put you away, Mrs Jolly. It's all right. Come on now.'

I led her back with her body racked with sobs, down the road to her house. Frank was waiting with the children standing in the lighted doorway.

'Is she OK, doctor?'

'Yes Frank, just played out.'

We put her to bed and I gave her a good dose of phenobarb from my bag. It was pretty well the only sedative we had at the time except chloral mixture or paraldehyde (which stinks atrociously), and I hadn't either of these anyway.

When she had settled down, I went to have a word with Frank. We sat at the kitchen table together. The picture was becoming very clear. I ought to have seen what was happenng before. Mrs Jolly's indomitability had always been a bit brittle. While Frank was stretching the family to the limit, she'd been using up her strength to keep things going, and all the time she had really been a mild manic depressive. She was now breaking out of the depressive phase that she'd been in since Frank's recovery and had gone wild.

I couldn't put it to him in nice psychiatric terminology, for that wouldn't get the piggy over the stile tonight anyway. I explained it all to Frank and he seemed to understand instinctively. She must have quiet, be given time, be cared for.

Frank turned up trumps. While we kept his wife under mild sedation, he got home from work early, made the evening meal, did the washing, brought home the shopping, and loved his wife in a practical, human way. After a time, she got off the swings and roundabouts of her mind and became a quieter, easier person.

Perhaps we should have anticipated it and taken precautions: eleven months later they had their fourth child after a gap of nine years. I was scared of her going into a puerperal depression – but happily she didn't. It was a beautiful baby, just beautiful. After all, they weren't a bad-looking couple, but this fair-haired, blue-eyed babe was positively angelic.

There ought to be a fairy-tale ending to this Jolly tale but there isn't. At four months, the baby wasn't doing the things it should. I was slow on the uptake again.

'She's not trying to get things, doctor.'

Mrs Jolly held a shiny rattle within arm's reach of the baby. She made no attempt to get hold of it. She didn't follow moving things with her eyes either. I waved my hands in front of her face. She never blinked. My heart missed a beat or two.

'Mrs Jolly . . .' I began.

'All right doctor, I know. I've guessed it for a week or two. Wendy's blind, isn't she?'

'Yes, Mrs Jolly, she is.'

We got the ophthalmologist to examine her. The terrible truth was that Mrs Jolly had had a bad delivery and she'd received excessive oxygen. This had caused an overgrowth of the blood vessels in the eye which had cut off Wendy's sight. This process wasn't properly understood at the time; all we knew was that she was blind.

Somehow the Jollys carried on, but when little Wendy could walk, she went to a special home for blind children where they had the expertise to teach her to overcome her disability. The Jollys saw her on every visiting day and she developed almost like a normal child.

I went round to see her when they had her home for the day. Frank watched her being taken round their back garden by the older children.

'Odd, ain't it, doctor? Wendy goes blind just as we're beginning to see.'

13
'Where my caravan has rested'

I think instinctively, 'I know that cough'. There is a knock on the door. 'Come in.' I am right – it's Mrs Blagdon. She is a tall, dark-skinned, handsome woman of about thirty-five, 'robus' as they say in Sussex.

'Hullo, Mrs Blagdon – sit down. Now tell me, what's the matter?' (I'll be very surprised if it isn't the usual.)

'It's me toobs, doctor.' I'm right again. 'Reel bronical I am; corf, corf – corf, corf, goes on all night. Can you give me something?'

I refrain from saying yet again, 'You really must cut down your smoking.' It's never produced any results in the past and unlikely to now.

I'm on the point of once more giving her a cough suppressant, maybe a new one to try, but none of them do any real good unless the patient helps himself. I stop, pen suspended over the prescription pad . . . Could she possibly be developing cancer? Chronic smokers do, without any real change in symptoms – I'd better make sure.

'Before I give you something for the cough, Mrs Blagdon, I think we'll just get an X-ray of your chest.'

Her eyes open wide.

'Are you worried about something, doctor? Do I need to?'

'Now, don't you worry, Mrs Blagdon, it'll just be good to know there's nothing much wrong, won't it?'

'If you say so, doctor. Don't fancy them 'ospitals meself.' She took the X-ray form reluctantly and got up.

'How's Willie getting on, Mrs Blagdon?'

'Oh, 'e's fine now doctor, 'is leg's 'ealed up luvly, fanks. Well, bye-bye now.'

'Willie' had needed a late call a month before. It had been so much out of the usual run of visits that I recalled every detail.

Miss Spencer had written, 'Willie Blagdon, 12a Downs Road', in the visiting book. I knew that '12a' usually meant someone superstitiously avoiding a '13', but as I drove along Downs Road I began to feel a bit irritated; there was 10, 11, 12, 14, 16 but no 12a *or* 13.

I reversed slowly down the road and then I saw the passageway between 12 and 14, more like a drive than a footpath, right between the tall, blank sides of the houses. I stopped the car, took my bag and walked down it.

All was revealed. At the back behind the houses was a wide paved yard, and in the yard stood a caravan. On its side in the fading light I could just read in crude scrawl '12a'.

This was no shining aluminium trailer but a real, old, gypsy, horse-drawn *Vaado* with yellow panels picked out in blue and scarlet, decorated wooden wheels and a rounded canvas-covered roof. Smoke spiralled into the air from a short black chimney-pipe, and at the end of the van a cosy yellow light shone through the lace curtains of the window in the top half of a stable-type door. A short flight of wooden steps ran up to it. I climbed two of them and tapped on the door.

The curtain was twitched aside and I heard a boy's voice.

'It's the croaker Ma, shall I open the jigger?'

'Open it, son.' It was Henrietta Blagdon's voice.

Both sections of the door opened and Mrs Blagdon stood in the doorway looking down at me rather like a queen, but her proud black eyes were welcoming. I felt as if an honour was being conferred on me when she said, 'Come inside, doctor.'

A whippet was poking out his nose suspiciously at me from under her skirt.

'Never you mind the jouk, doctor,' she said. ' 'E won't 'urt a fly.'

Many of the gypsies that used to travel the roads of the south of England had given up the losing battle with the traffic and the hostility of farmers and had settled in houses in the towns. It looked as if the Blagdons had done the same, only they'd brought their home with them. Tucked away here in this yard they had a semblance of their old life. I imagine the council had turned a blind eye to their 'substandard' accommodation. It meant one less on the housing list.

Charles had warned me that few of the true Romanies trusted the Health Service. They preferred to pay – the medicine couldn't be much good if it were free.

'You'll find what they think you're worth tucked under an ornament on the mantelpiece,' he'd told me. 'You take it without a word and then the contract is fixed. They've paid you and you've undertaken to do your best, no matter what.'

It was even as he had said: there, beneath a copper-lustreware jug, protruded the corner of paper currency. I got wise to my estimated value when I found it was a ten-shilling note. However, according to protocol, I slipped it into my pocket without a word, and turned to Henrietta.

'What's wrong with Willie then?' I inquired.

We were all standing close together in the limited space of the van. She pointed down and I followed her finger to Willie's leg. It was bandaged from foot to knee, rather expertly I thought.

'What happened to him then?'

'Well doctor, I just sent 'im over the tober for ten-pennoth o' sawney, I mean, acrost the road for tenpence-worf of bacon.' (This was when tenpence, old money, would buy

92

enough bacon for a family dinner and not just the wrapping.) 'Along come this woman wearin' a comic 'at, an' Willie, 'e looks back at me an' 'ollers, "Dic at the molisher ma, wiv 'at caster on 'er nob!", when round the corner comes a moty-car an' knocks the li'l chavvy inter the gutter.

'Wasn't the driver's fault but yet I couldn't 'ardly blime Willie neither, it was that old girl in 'er perishin' 'at. Got a bloomin' great cut on 'is leg, 'e 'as, so I done 'im up best I could an' calls you, doctor.'

Willie winced as I undid the bandage but he never uttered a sound, which wasn't bad for a lad of eight. He had a nasty three-inch gash on the shin, but the edges of the wound were nicely together and I didn't fancy giving Willie more pain with stitches, so I cleaned it with dilute antiseptic and put new dressings on it.

'When your husband comes home, Mrs Blagdon, bring Willie down to the surgery and we'll give him a tetanus injection. I know he had the first ones when he was a baby – he'll only need one.'

Willie's ankle was badly bruised but there were no bones broken, so I said, 'He ought to rest it after this for a few days, and I'll get a nurse to come in and re-do the bandages.'

Mrs Blagdon looked a bit hurt.

'Thought I done it up nice, doctor.'

'Yes, fine, Mrs Blagdon, but we'd better get it checked, hadn't we?'

I looked down at the boy. 'You'd better look both ways next time, old son.'

At that moment the door opened and in came Josiah, Henrietta's husband.

'Evenin' doctor,' then, ' 'Ullo, young chavlo, what you done to yerself? Bin in a scrap, 'ave yer? Told yer last time I'd put you on bread an' water if yer did.'

'Oh stop yer patter, Jos,' cut in Mrs Blagdon. 'It was a moty-car what done it!'

'Sorry then, son,' Josiah put his hand on the boy's head and ruffled his dark hair, then he subsided into one of the two miniature armchairs by the stove.

It wasn't difficult to see who wore the trousers. Josiah

didn't have the looks of a true Romany. I got the impression that this put him at a disadvantage, but Henrietta's dark eyes would have quelled a doughtier spirit. He looked, anyway, a quiet man. As he sat there there was a curious, dreamy quality about him.

'Stop for a cupper tea, doctor?' Henrietta had her hand up to the gaily-painted tea-caddy on the shelf above the little glowing range on which a kettle had been quietly steaming. I noticed the ornate gold and silver rings glinting on her fingers in the lamplight. She was already filling the brown shiny teapot. 'Don't mind if I do, thank you.'

While the tea was brewing, Josiah went out to feed the pony. I had heard the clip-clop just before he came in and the rattle of his cart. He was a 'totter' – a rag-and-bone man. 'Does all right for us, doctor, even though 'e can't read nor write.' Henrietta looked after her man with a smile of affection.

'How on earth does he manage?' I asked.

She smiled again. 'Don't need no bank for 'is money, doctor, but 'e knows a bob from a tanner any day. Besides, I 'elps 'im. My dad put me to school; wherever we was stoppin' a spell, off to school I 'ad to go or 'e'd wallop me. Got quite a bit o' book learnin'. Any'ow . . .' She said something in Romany which could have been Sanskrit so far as I was concerned, and probably *was*, more or less.

'Tell me what that means, Mrs Blagdon,' I said.

'The bee get 'oney from flowers,' she answered with a sly grin. 'Jos knows where to go for 'is money.' She paused. 'I'll tell you something else, doctor, which might surprise yer.'

She crossed the van in one stride and opened the door of a neat little built-in cupboard. 'Look in 'ere, doctor.'

There was an old portable gramophone and a small pile of records. I picked up the top ones and read the label: 'Dvořák, New World Symphony. First movement.' I turned over more – all Dvořák.

' 'E picked up the old grammerphone and them records at a farmhouse what 'ad cleared 'em out alongside a lot of junk. 'E played that top record when 'e got 'ome. Funny! Never seed 'im like it before; all dreamy-like. Said it made 'im think of the old times on the road, cookin' fires an' that. In the end 'e played the lot an' 'e often does. Funny old Moush, my Jos.' Her eyes were bright as though they weren't far from tears.

She handed me a fine Crown Derby cup, with just one small chip in the saucer, and I drank my tea in silence. I was just a bit amazed. Here was a gypsy without formal education, responding instinctively to classical music, perhaps caught by the folk themes in the 'New World'.

I glanced around the small interior of the caravan for any further clues to explain this phenomenon. Most was typical of a Romany mobile dwelling. A basket hung over the door; brass and copper jugs, all highly polished, stood on the mantelshelf, china ornaments behind a guard-rail on a tiny side cabinet. The far end was filled by a built-in bed with curtains part-drawn and a cupboard bed underneath, evidently where Willie kipped. Pillows and sheets, such as were visible, were edged with lace.

Pictures crowded the walls. Mostly they were of religious sentimentality, children, unhealthily virtuous-looking, crossing broken bridges over raging torrents while, hovering unseen above their heads, angels guarded their charges. But there were one or two surprises. Two small watercolours that looked like Lamorna Birch, and a print of horses by Dame Laura Knight. Henrietta was following my eyes.

'Picked 'em up on 'is tottin'. Wouldn't part wiv 'em agin though.'

Jos was certainly an unusual gypsy. He came in from his pony, sat down on the other chair again and drank with audible relish.

'Could do with that,' he said. 'Proper cold on that old cart – not like your nice warm car, doctor.'

I came to with a jerk. 'Better be getting on my way; thanks for the tea. Now look after that leg of Willie's. See you at the surgery.'

The cut healed well, and Henrietta's X-ray, thankfully, was clear and the Blagdons passed out of my life for several months.

It was late one morning when a phone call was put through to me.

'Dr Hamilton? Sister Miller, Ward 4, Duke of Gloucester. Sorry you haven't been notified before. It's about Josiah Blagdon; he came through casualty a week ago. Compound fracture of tib and fib, lower third. That's not the trouble, it's in good position. It's Mr Blagdon himself. He's withdrawn, doesn't read anything or talk to the other patients, and he is just not eating. I really am worried. He won't do well like this. I wondered whether you as his doctor had any special line on him?'

'I'll come and see him this afternoon, sister.'

'Thank you, doctor, I'd be most grateful.'

I found the sister in her little room.

'By the way, sister, perhaps no one's said, you know he can't read.'

'Oh dear, that explains part of it,' she said. 'I should have twigged it. His wife signed all the papers.'

'Well, don't let him know I told you.'

Jos was in a bed at the far end of the ward where the windows look out to the Downs. I came up quietly and for a moment he didn't seem to notice who I was. His eyes had the peculiar look of a trapped animal – trapped, with no way it could see to escape.

'Hullo, Jos.' I felt I could presume to call him that.

His eyes focussed like a man just waking, then he grinned and stuck out a hand. 'Hullo, doc! Fancy you coming to see me!'

'Oh we quite often do, just to see you're behaving yourselves. How did all this happen then?'

'Didn't you see, doctor? Missus said it was in the local paper.'

'No Jos – tell me.'

'Well, it wus like this. I was goin' down the 'ill to the 'arbour when the pony shied at a cat runnin' across the road, the old wheel 'its the kerb an' over we goes. 'Aven't felt so good in 'ere, like bein' in stir – not that I 'ave bin, don't fancy me grub, can't get me kip, reckon I need me missus an' me kid . . .'

'And the fresh air and the tober,' I added, and he grinned. 'Well Jos, you'll be out of here in no time. What about cheering up some of these blokes?' (I waved my hand round the ward.) 'Some are here for the duration. Tell 'em about your totting.'

'OK doc, I'll try.'

'Got to go now.' I shook his hand. 'And, one thing more, if the sister tells me you're not eating *all* your grub – I'll come and stuff it down your throat with my bare hands!'

He grinned again and waved his hand as I went off down the ward. As I reached sister's door, I had a crazy idea. I asked her to get the hospital network to play part of Dvořak's 'New World', and to make sure that Jos was listening on his headphones.

Jos began to mend and was discharged in the minimum time, and it wasn't long before he was back totting again. Some of his mates had salvaged his cart and Henrietta had been well up to caring for the pony, with Willie's help. Once again I forgot about Jos until, in the autumn, a big bag of beautiful chestnuts mysteriously found their way on to our doorstep.

In the spring we decided to take a leaf out of his book. We bought a second-hand caravan of our own – not a horse-drawn one, but quite a nice towing one with calor gas, just big enough to take the lot of us. It would give us marvellously cheap family holidays, maybe a week at a time, which was about as long as we could stand each other at such close quarters.

We found a beautiful quiet spot on a farm only ten miles from Wilverton, on a lower slope of the north side of the Downs. The farmer was very kind – he didn't know us yet! There was almost every mod con. The field he showed us had a stand-pipe to a water trough in the corner, there was a wood nearby on the Downs with an abundance of firewood and we were already accomplished loo-diggers.

We couldn't wait to get away. The school holidays were just coming up for Peter and Sarah. I decided to ask the partners, off the cuff, for time off.

'Well, you might give us more warning next time,' said

Charles. 'But it will be OK, we can cope. After all, you don't do all that much, do you?' He straightened my tie and picked a piece of fluff off my jacket. I let it pass; he's bigger than me.

There was still light in the sky as we set off late on the Friday. The lockers in the van were stuffed with packets and tins and we'd got half a dozen early lettuces from the crazy lean-to greenhouse. We stuffed cushions in the crockery cupboards to stop things getting broken. The afternoon rain had stopped and it was a beautiful clear evening.

An hour later, we were backing the van through the gateway into the field. Peter was holding the gate and Elisabeth giving instructions. Backing a trailer entails turning the steering wheel in the opposite direction to the way you usually do, at least, I thought so.

'Right-hand down a bit, now left – *stop*!'

But I was too late. There was a crunch and we'd stopped all right, but with the van over at a sickening angle. I leapt out. Sarah was crying, 'Our lovely van'. The offside wheel had gone round a large stone half-buried in the grass and the sub-axle had snapped off.

Our mobile home was no longer mobile; we were stuck fast and, what was more, slap in the gateway of Farmer Elphick's field. I walked down to the farmer to tell him of the predicament. He was quite accommodating.

'You'll be all right there till Monday; not ready to put the sheep in the top field.'

'I'll get it moved by then,' I said hopefully.

When I got back, we carefully wound down the van legs and got it fairly level. Elisabeth had sent the children to the wood a hundred yards away to get sticks. We called them back as it was getting dusk and began to cook a meal of baked beans and scrambled eggs on the calor stove, the gas-lamp giving us a cosy light.

As we were having our supper Elisabeth said, 'It's too late to put the tent up now. We'd all better scrum down in the van.'

'Oh goody!' said Sarah.

'Bags I the seat,' said Peter.

'You'll just go where you fit in best,' said Elisabeth, who wasn't going to have any monkeying around in that confined space. 'Barney, if you're a good boy, you can go on the floor with Sarah.'

'I be a good boy, Mummy,' said Barnaby, feeling it a privilege.

'You'd better be. I'm not having you jumping all over me,' said Sarah.

'All right, while you two get ready, Peter and I will do the washing-up outside. Come on, Pete.'

I lit a hurricane-lamp and carried out the water that had been heating on the stove while we'd been eating. A mist was rising and the stars were bright in the cold sky. Over at the edge of the wood a tawny owl hooted – I know it was a tawny owl, because Peter told me.

'Dad, this *is* fun – but what about the van axle?'

'Don't know, Peter, we'll have to see about that in the morning.'

'Suppose we're stuck here for ever?' Peter didn't sound as if that prospect worried him over much.

'We'll think of something.' But I wasn't sure what.

The van seemed very snug when we handed in the dishes. The other two were in their blanket sleeping-bags, side by side, heads to toes on the floor. We trod carefully by them. Washing and teeth-cleaning went by the board that night. Peter undressed sitting on his seat and got into his bag.

We had a little family prayer together before I turned off the gaslight and went to close the valve on the gas cylinder outside on the towing bracket. The children were really tired and in spite of the excitement they were soon asleep. I opened one window a little at the stove end and screwed the catch tight.

Elisabeth and I talked for a while in whispers.

'It'll bust the bank to get a breakdown crew and a truck out here,' I said.

'What about your friend Jos – the totter?' Elisabeth was having one of her brainwaves. 'He's got all sorts of connections – goes to breakers' yards and things. Couldn't he help us?'

'Hey – that's an idea. I'll see what's what in the morning.'

It was pretty cramped but we slept – well, some of the time.

Peter and Sarah went down to the farm soon after it was light. Their day had already begun down there, and the children came back with some milk and a bag of eggs. I got a little fire going with the sticks we'd kept free from dew under the van. We had porridge and milk, boiled eggs and rather dusky toast made by Peter over the fire. Then I set off in the car. I drove straight back to Wilverton and got to Downs Road, at twenty past eight. Jos was just harnessing his pony for a day's totting.

I gave him a quick run-down on our situation.

'Jos, do you think you could help us?'

He frowned. 'Can't promise nothin' – but I knows someone who breaks cars, don't know if 'e's any caravan axles though. 'Ave to see.'

I gave him the phone number of the farm and drove slowly back still wondering if we could get the van to rights somehow.

Mr Elphick told us it was their turn for morning service on the Sunday. The vicar had three other parishes to care for. So, after breakfast, we tidied ourselves up and walked down the road past the farm to the little church which lay, half-hidden, in a fold of the hill.

It was a quiet, grey building, confidently supporting an unusual round tower, the like of which I'd only seen before in Norfolk. The farmer – who combined his usual work with being churchwarden – had evidently just cut the grass with a scythe, as it lay in neat swaths by the path, all the way from the lych-gate to the porch. The pulpit was dark brown with intricate carving and obviously Jacobean, and only raised the preacher two feet above the congregation (quite high enough). When he got up into it and announced his subject, 'Mobilization', Elisabeth dug me in the ribs, but it was about the army of the church and not about caravans!

The closing hymn declared that 'Like a mighty army moves the church of God', and we marched out into the spring sunshine and the smell of cut grass, passing the vicarage cat which had been asleep in the pew behind us throughout the entire service.

We spent the afternoon wandering on the Downs with Barney walking most of the way. Peter thought he saw a raven but I told him rather unkindly that the last raven had been observed many years before. We went to bed full of fresh air and more baked beans.

Next day, we started off cleaning up the campsite. Peter and Sarah went off to the copse to collect firewood and we rigged up a stick-table outside the van to dry the crockery. Then we called them to come for elevenses.

We were sitting round drinking our coffee when we heard it. 'Clip, clop, clip, clop'. It was coming from behind the knoll where the flinty tract wound down to the farm and the village road. Then Jos's pony came in sight, pulling the cart, with Jos at the reins – and inside was a rusty but serviceable caravan axle.

'Got it for thirty bob, doctor,' said Jos smiling.

He'd brought some tools as well. We lifted the caravan higher on its legs and unfixed the axle. Jos helped us get the replacement attached. Then we stood back to admire our work.

'Now then Jos, what do we owe you?'

'Thirty bob, doctor.'

'Come on, Jos, what about your profit, your time and your labour?'

'Thirty bob,' he said, 'or I takes it off again. I seem to remember someone comin' to see me in 'ospital an' gettin' a record played for me on the phones. I know – sister tipped me off. This is a kind o' thank you.'

But for Jos, my caravan might still be resting in that farm gateway on the other side of the Downs.

14

Peter

His first term's report said, 'Peter is trying'. The second, 'Peter is still trying'. We felt that at any rate he was holding his own, if not advancing. The third term's report said, 'Peter is rather trying'. By this time we realized he wasn't doing very well at school, and Elisabeth and I got concerned about it.

It was a year now since he had started at this school. It seemed as if he just couldn't make good the lack of teaching he'd suffered in Africa, and was getting fed up into the bargain. Elisabeth, who is a first-rate Froebel teacher, had had his early years' education all planned out. It all went haywire with her prolonged ill-health abroad, and Pete was only too happy to be out with his beloved birds and beasts rather than stuck indoors with books.

We felt we owed it to him to give him the extra help he needed now. We were doctors to Hillside Grange, a small boarding school in the Downs behind the town. Although it seemed crazy to spend money on boarding him out when we lived nearby, the standards of teaching and discipline were so good that we felt we must bust ourselves to get him there.

The fees were £65 a term, so we said goodbye to a stair-carpet and new curtains for an indefinite period and booked him for the autumn term. Sarah was getting along very nicely in her little school, so we weren't so concerned about her.

Nevertheless, the family didn't look forward to the start of term. Peter for his part viewed the prospect with equanimity, even with pleasurable anticipation – in fact he was rarin' to go! In spite of his love of wandering around the countryside, he is a gregarious young animal, and the thought of having a constant supply of cronies of his own age obviously gave him a great deal of satisfaction.

There was something solid and comforting about that

school building. Hillside Grange had been a private house in the 'spacious days' of Wilverton. Although only about a hundred years old, Hillside had somehow avoided the banal, over-elaborated clumsiness of a typical Victorian country house. By blending Kentish rag stone and mellow Sussex brick and contenting himself with a long low building of two main storeys and a few dormers in the roof, the architect had produced a pleasing and well-balanced structure that warmed rather than depressed the eye. The mullioned windows were not out of place even though they were out of period. You felt it would be easy to be happy there.

'Goodbye Peter, do your best, see you soon.'

'Bye, Daddy.'

I looked down at the sturdy nine-year-old, dressed in his new grey suit and red and white tie. Perhaps it would be more honest to say 'nearly new grey suit'. Buying all that kit on a school list had been prohibitively expensive. We had had to resort to the school store, where hard-up parents like us could buy part-worn or out-grown clothes which the parents of other boys had returned. As it all came from Harrods, it was pretty hard-wearing stuff.

I'll say this for Pete, he never raised objections to wearing second-hand clobber. He looked up at me now and smiled a little wanly, for all his erstwhile zest at going to boarding school. He held out his hand. I restrained an almost over-powering impulse to give him a hug, and solemnly shook it instead. It would never have done to show emotion; there were a bunch of small faces peering curiously through the bay window at the side of the big front door of the school and Pete would have been ragged unmercifully, I am sure, if I'd given in to my feelings.

He turned and pushed open the tall oak doors and they swung shut behind him. I gave my nose a good blow on the way back to the car.

'For goodness' sake,' I told myself. 'What are you getting sentimental about? The boy will be approximately one mile away and you'll see him on Sunday anyway.' Still . . . it *was* the first time he'd really been away from home.

'All boys will write home once a week.' That's what the

school brochure stated. Sure enough on Wednesday, Peter's letter arrived. It showed a mixture of pride and pique.

'Dear Mummy and Daddy,
     'It is sooper here.' ('Little blighter, he doesn't miss us at all,' said Elisabeth.) 'I got the sliper yesterday. I had just mad my bed when James Mi muked it up.
He is a roter, I got blamed for it but I dident sneek on him.'

Elisabeth made sympathetic clucking noises and wrote one or two kind things back but I added a postscript: 'Bad luck about the slippering but it will teach you not to expect justice in this world, old chap, and, by the way, slipper has two "p's".'

We duly attended school chapel on Sunday and Peter came home for a half day. He was allowed two chocolate biscuits for tea instead of one, in spite of protests from Barney, as he had to be back soon after tea.

It was about eight in the evening when I was on call the following week that I got a telephone message from the assistant school matron. She was a bright, round-faced girl, doing a year after being a ward sister at the Middlesex Hospital, before getting married. Matron, who was older and had been with the school for half her lifetime, was off duty that night.

'Doctor, I'm worried about one boy. He's had a rigor and he's got quite a high temperature. Could you come and see him?'

I found the little chap, Higginson, curiously brown-looking, considering the summer we'd had. He was very hot and complaining of a terrible headache and backache. He seemed slightly delirious in the way he answered questions. Apart from a temperature of 104° there wasn't much else to go on.

'He only came back from seeing his parents in Nigeria a week ago,' the assistant matron told me.

The penny dropped – *that* was why he was so sunburnt and, almost certainly, that was also why he was so acutely ill. I took some blood and rang up for an emergency laboratory examination at the Duke of Gloucester's.

An hour later the pathologist rang back: 'The blood is full of parasites – definitely malaria.'

We got a chemist out from his flat above his shop and a master went down and collected some mepacrine. In a few days, Higginson was feeling perfectly well; however we continued treatment for several weeks to make sure we'd eradicated the infection as far as possible.

I was coming down the big oak stairs from the school sanatorium where I'd just given Higginson permission to go back to classes, when Rickards came out of his study in the hall. Rickards was the headmaster of Hillside.

'Ah, doctor, nice to see you. All well up there? I've been waiting for an opportunity to have a chat; could you spare me a minute?'

We went into the room where books and papers vied for space with footballs, squash rackets and hockey sticks.

'It's about Peter. I know it's early days, but his form master has had a chance to size him up a bit. He has got seriously behind in the basics, hasn't he? That's not the real problem, however. He seems to lack incentive. It's almost as if he hasn't had a chance to succeed at anything yet. If he could, I think his work and everything else would improve.'

I felt this was a bit of a snap judgement on poor old Peter as he'd only been there such a short time, but Rickards was a good man with lots of experience.

I thought about Peter's success in bird-watching but that seemed a little way out – not exactly a competitive exercise, you might say – although to listen to some bird-watchers you could be forgiven for thinking it was.

There wasn't much opportunity to do anything about Peter immediately following this conversation as the whole school suffered a major set-back. One boy began complaining of sickness and then went yellow; soon there was wave after wave of boys going down like ninepins with infectious jaundice. Fortunately it was of a mild variety, but with almost half the school down at any one time plus several of the staff, it took the stuffing out of the school curriculum and set us back quite a bit in our practice programme as well.

But it had its moments. As we were doing a 'ward round'

with matron, who was too hard-bitten to succumb to such a miserable little virus, we reached a bed whose occupant was a diminutive, dark-skinned boy. Matron was under considerable pressure, as was understandable, and hadn't mastered all the new boys' names in her usual meticulous way. She glanced at her list of patients.

'What's your name, sonny?' she asked quickly.

The whites of his eyes enlarged in his sultry countenance. He sprang to his feet and stood erect on his bed, his head just level with my chest.

'I am Prince ——.'

He was indeed – the younger brother of the ruler of a Middle Eastern state and his dignity had been wounded.

'All right, you can lie down again,' said matron.

When we were outside the room she added, 'I spend half my time answering phone calls from London, from the ambassador of his country wanting to know if the boy's seen a specialist and so on.'

At that moment the telephone rang in her office. It was another call from the embassy.

'Let me deal with it,' I whispered. 'This is Doctor Hamilton here. Yes, Prince —— is doing very well. No, he is not in any danger. No, he does not need to see a specialist. No, it is not possible for him to be visited now, he is probably still infectious, but I expect he will be able to resume his studies in a few days. Yes, if the headmaster agrees you may see him then. Now I have other patients to attend to. If you care to telephone in a week's time . . . Thank you. Goodbye.'

I turned to the matron. 'I hope that will give you a bit of peace now.'

She grinned. 'Some hope – but thanks.'

On my way down the stairs I met Rickards again – this seemed to be becoming a habit. He had more of a suppliant look in his eye this time; perhaps the epidemic at the school was wearing him down.

'Hamilton, I believe you were a boxing blue,' he commenced abruptly, but in an unusually reverential tone.

'Yes,' I answered. 'I was.'

'I don't suppose you would care to give some tuition to

the boys, would you? At a time of your own choosing, of course.'

I wondered how on earth I could fit it in – this was a busy time of year for us – but I couldn't resist it.

'I think I could. What about Thursday evenings?'

Thursday was my half day – I hoped Elisabeth would understand.

'That would be splendid,' Rickards beamed.

Our coach at Cambridge, Bill Child, three times ABA light heavyweight champion in his day, had inculcated some sound principles of the 'noble art' into the boxing team. I racked my brains now, as to how I could adapt his routine for small boys.

On Thursday, I found about sixteen boys of assorted sizes, from minute to small, all fitted with enormous boxing gloves and positively lusting to pulverize their best friends. I'm sure their ferocity would have shocked their mothers' tender hearts.

We started by getting some discipline and order into the proceedings.

First I stood them in line and, unless left-handed, they all put their left foot forward; if left-handed, they had to put their right foot forward. I demonstrated how to advance and retire with the boxer's shuffle; having absorbed this, they were taught to guard with the right and to deliver a straight left, at the word of command. Occasionally they were allowed the luxury of a follow-up with the right – the old 'one two'.

After a time I paired them off according to size, and allowed a minute of controlled sparring. One after another they had to break off to spar with me to learn the principle of slipping a left lead and of hitting cleanly with a properly closed glove.

Peter had joined the squad on his own accord. At last it came to his turn to spar with me.

'Now then, Peter, I want you to lead with your left at my face.'

I planned to dodge as usual, to show how speed of punch was necessary, but the words weren't out of my mouth before he landed a perfect straight left, with the kick of at least a small mule, slap on my nose. Tears streamed down my cheeks and a trickle of blood dripped from my nose. I wiped it on my sleeve. You can't wipe your nose with a handkerchief with boxing gloves on.

'Oh sir,' said Peter anxiously. 'Have I hurt you?'

'That's OK. Good punch,' I grunted.

I'm sure the psychologists would explain that some inhibiting parental image was removed from Peter's mind at that moment. Whatever it was – from then on Peter very quickly became a first-rate boxer for his age and, more important, his work improved by leaps and bounds.

Perhaps Rickards had got it right. Peter needed to succeed at something – even boxing would do. As the weeks went by, I realized that not only was Rickards extremely adept at getting the best out of the boys – he was no slouch at getting what he wanted out of parents too.

The boxing class was proving quite successful. It was spurred on by a demonstration I organized. One of our patients was a leader of a local boys' club, boxing section. A protégé of his was runner-up in the ABA Junior Championships at middleweight, and he kindly came and gave a demonstration with one of his pals from the club.

Rickards now focussed his persuasive wiles on my most vulnerable spot.

The jaundice epidemic was at last clearing up, and he invited me to have a cup of coffee in his sanctum one morning. Through the window a homogeneous mass of boys in red and white hooped jerseys were sweeping this way and that across a field, rather like a flock of coloured starlings, pursued by a harassed mistress with a whistle. Small rugby posts stood at each end.

'Hamilton, we're in trouble again. Both the rugger masters are down with jaundice as you know. Poor Miss Peckton isn't cut out for the game; could you possibly spare an odd hour to teach them the elements? I know it is asking a lot but you have had such a success with the boxing.'

A few well-chosen words of flattery achieved his purpose.

'Of course, I'd love to. What about starting now?' I pointed out of the window.

'My dear chap – you're not clad for it.'

'Not to worry,' I said, doffing my jacket and tucking my trousers in my socks. 'Have you got an old sweater you could lend me?'

He fished one out of a drawer and handed it to me.

'Try this.'

'Right, half an hour today only,' and I ran out on to the field.

Miss Peckton gladly surrendered her whistle to me and stood watching on the touch-line.

We separated the two teams, assembled the heavier boys in two five-man scrums and arranged the backs in the positions they looked most suitable to fill.

It was not the time for a lot of skills' development or accurate learning of rules, but they needed to learn something about keeping to positions at least and how to pass the ball and, above all, to have some fun and enjoy it.

It was pretty chaotic but enjoy it they did. I played alternately on either side, keeping little movements going. I offered sixpence to any boy who would tackle me. Quickly I'd promised forth all my spare cash.

Half an hour later, having scrubbed my hands in the head's own cloakroom, I set out for my last two routine visits. I was a little embarrassed when I noticed the companion of one patient pointedly opening the window as I left. I *was* a bit high after all that running, I suppose.

Rickards' next ploy for getting parental assistance was very much off the cuff. I cannot accuse him of any premeditation but his psychology and timing were perfect nevertheless. He played upon my finer feelings with the touch of an artist.

Elisabeth, Sarah, Barney and I were in loyal attendance at the school's chapel service one Sunday morning. As the clock hands moved round to five to ten, the reverential hush was broken by a growing whispering. Heads began to turn towards the door. Rickards was on the edge of his chair in the back row where we sat with other parents.

At ten o'clock, when we should have begun the service, he came over and whispered in my ear.

'Would you come out for a minute, doctor?'

Outside in the hall he spoke rapidly.

'Hamilton, forgive me, I know I have trespassed on your good will before, but obviously the vicar isn't coming – we must have got our wires crossed somehow. You were a missionary, weren't you? Could you possibly take the service for us – as a great favour? It's a straight run – I've marked the passages in the Prayer Book and the hymns are on a sheet on the lectern. I would be very much obliged if you would undertake it.'

I thought quickly. This was definitely a one-off situation for me, but it would be an opportunity, apart from not letting Rickards down in front of the parents – an opportunity for ordinary things like football and fun to be linked in the minds of the boys with the most important thing of all, the friendship of Jesus.

'Give me a minute to nip out to my car,' I whispered.

'Right, I'll just announce that you are kindly going to conduct the service.'

As I walked down to the front, I felt parental eyes on me. Curious? Hostile? Who was this guy acting as preacher? But I knew dear Elisabeth was thinking of me.

When I turned to face the assembled company, my embarrassment simply evaporated. Change the colour of their faces and their clothes, and they were just another congregation such as I had often enjoyed speaking to in Africa.

The service, though I say it myself, went with quite a swing! I think just possibly there was slightly less solemnity than normal about it and we cut a few corners.

Then we came to the talk. I stood up.

'What's this?' I asked the boys, and produced from my pocket the rubber glove I'd got from the car. It hung limp and empty from my fingers. Half a dozen boys said:

'A rubber glove.'

One older one ventured:

'A surgeon's glove.'

'Right – what do you use it for?'

'Operations, sir.'

'Yes, but it's no use like this, is it?' I wagged it in the air.

110

'How about it now?' I blew it up and held it swollen and looking like a fat hand. 'It looks better, but will it work?'

'No sir,' they chorused.

I turned my back and slipped it on.

'Now then, what can it do now?' I picked up a pencil, with my gloved hand.

'Now the glove can *do* things – it's useful. If it's sterilized, it can do wonderful operations. Some of us are like rubber gloves, limp and floppy, people can flip us around any old way, we're not much use to anybody. But some of us are like a blown-up glove. We look more or less all right – but really we're only puffed up with our own ideas. When it comes to real action, like helping people who are in need, we are powerless. We are all show. What do we really need, we human gloves?'

Words from the back.

'We need a hand in it, sir.'

'Right, we need a hand – and not just any old hand, but a strong, kind hand, an expert's hand like a surgeon's hand. We need Jesus' hand in our lives. Jesus told parables, didn't he? Parables are stories to help us understand things about God. What I've just told you is a parable – the story of a glove. The glove represents you and me. We need to let Jesus put his hand into our lives – his strong hand, his kind hand, his expert hand. Let him grip us, then he'll be in control and help us to do things that are really worthwhile, things that we couldn't do ourselves, like overcoming what's wrong in our lives and doing right. The apostle Paul said: "I can do all things through Christ who strengthens me." He found that it was true – that when Jesus gripped his life he became strong.'

We sang the last hymn and I said a closing prayer.

On the way out Rickards gripped my arm.

'Thank you, doctor. You've given us something to think about.'

News travels fast on the scholastic grape-vine. Before the end of term, Springmount, a rival school a mile or two away, for whom our practice also provided medical care and attention, had word of my pugilistic past. Their headmaster rang me up at the end of surgery one morning.

'I wonder if you would be free to referee our school boxing championships. We're holding them next Thursday afternoon.'

The grape-vine *had* been working well. They even knew my afternoon off, but then, perhaps they knew that anyway. Once again I gave way and duly appeared at the ring-side table, with a list of contestants and a timekeeper with a small electric bell.

All I can remember of the method of point-scoring is that a point is registered for blows on the 'target', which is upwards from the waist (not counting the arms), and they must be delivered with the knuckle part of the glove. If the points are equal, skill in attack and defence must be taken into account. I didn't need to watch the whirlwind of small arms and bodies for more than one bout to realize that I'd better judge the winner on my general impression and hope for the best. I felt a new respect for the skill of referees in major contests.

All went well and everyone seemed happy until the second to last bout. Two small, handsome, dark-haired boys climbed into the ring, their golden-brown skin and almond eyes revealing their Eastern origin. I was getting used to royalty now, and was only mildly impressed when told that one was a prince and the other the son of one of his nobles.

But I was quite unprepared for the bout that followed. The prince attacked his opponent with enormous zest, while the miniature nobleman defended himself with the utmost skill and agility, leaping round the ring in reverse, ducking, parrying and side-stepping, but never laying a glove on his attacker.

The one-minute rounds came quickly to an end. Neither had landed a punch, but as the prince had done all the attacking, I had to give him the verdict. This afforded him great satisfaction and, strangely enough, it just seemed to be a relief to his opponent. I badly wanted to know more about these two lads, but evening surgery was due, so my questions had to remain unasked, and later they were simply forgotten in the rush of daily life.

The years went by and one evening I was attending a post-graduate lecture at the Duke of Gloucester Hospital. I found myself sitting at supper before the lecture next to a young doctor who had just returned from the East, in fact, from the very homeland of my two young pugilists from the past.

'How did you find the country?' I asked.

'Great opportunities for medical advance,' he said. 'But it's going through a period of change now that the old king is dead and his son has taken over.'

'D'you know, I once refereed a boxing match between the new king and one of his nobles, when they were boys.'

He laughed. 'Don't tell me – I can guess who won!'

'Well, who did?'

'The prince, of course – my dear chap, it was more than that other little lad's life was worth to lay a finger on his sovereign – he is regarded as semi-divine, you know!'

I felt that some master at Springmount should have got wise to that fact before matching them.

At Hillside Grange, the rugby master returned to his coaching and I retired gracefully although I occasionally helped out when asked. I was very keen to see how the first team progressed however. Their principal fixture was with a Brighton school. They were to play at home.

When the great day arrived, I found myself on the touch-line next door to the visitors' headmaster. To his great chagrin his team, normally invincible, was being given a run-around by Hillside Grange. I got quite carried away and bellowed encouragement whenever our home team had the ball. In the end Hillside won by just two points. I felt generous in victory, though why *I* felt so victorious I don't know.

As we walked off I said to him cheerily, 'Sorry if I shouted rather a lot – got a bit enthused, you know!'

'Filthy noise,' he growled and strode off to sit gloomily in the bus until his team, who were far less disgruntled than he, had had their tea.

'Not to mind. Takes it all a bit too seriously,' Rickards murmured in my ear as I munched my currant bun in the hall with the boys.

15
Exeat

Sarah and Barney were cavorting about on the grass. It wasn't doing their shoes or the grass much good. Elisabeth and I stood in the school drive waiting for Peter to 'demerge', as Sarah would have put it. One small boy after another came out, sedately at first, red cap in hand; then, sticking it on his head, he would rush exuberantly to his parents, to be carried off for a blissful Sunday *exeat*. At last a familiar face with chubby pink cheeks and large, brown, cow-like eyes appeared.

'Hullo, Mum. Hullo, Dad.' He allowed Mum to give him a kiss but not Dad, and then, collecting the muddy Sarah and Barney, off we went in the Volkswagen.

For an English March, it was a glorious day. The landscape was sodden with weeks of rain but the sky was blue, and a yellow sun, hanging low on the horizon, still shone quite warmly on the countryside.

Up the Downs road we hurried, through the little upland valleys and down into the weald beyond. This was where we would see the birds in the copses and by the streams. It was, after all, Peter's day, so birds it had to be.

There had been a kestrel hovering in the breeze above our heads as we breasted the Downs. Even as we spotted it, it stooped to fall like a brown star into the bracken. Peter looked back through the rear window. He saw it come back up with something in its claws.

'Probably a vole,' he commented in knowledgeable tones. We found a quiet road running through a wood. Blackbirds were singing aggressively as they marked out their territory. A jay cackled off among the trees as we stopped the car in a roadside space at the bottom of the wood. We walked back down the road to where a white barred bridge crossed the stream full with rain-water. Sarah was towing Barney by the hand and chattering.

'Sh, sh,' hissed Peter. 'You'll never see anything.'

Though we were quiet as we approached the bridge, we started a heron down by the stream.

'Catching minnows,' said Elisabeth, who knows more about nature than any of us, as the heron flapped ponderously away across the field and landed at a safe distance a hundred yards off.

Peter and I watched him through binoculars. First, he stood very straight and tall, watching for danger. Reassured, he folded his neck in an S bend, lifted one leg up under the tummy and relaxed. Then the fun began. A pair of crows winged over from the trees by the stream, resenting this large intruder in their field. Both dive-bombed the heron, wheeling in from different sides: one banked up into the tree and the other taxied to a halt a few yards behind the heron. He merely looked round disdainfully.

We could hear the crows talking. We could imagine the conversation. The one in the tree, feeling well out of reach of the heron's spear, was saying, 'Go on mate, 'ave a go – see 'im orf, 'e don't belong 'ere!'

The other, to show he didn't care how big the heron was, began sidling up behind him, pecking at the ground.

The heron's head slowly revolved backwards at 180° but he made no other move. When the crow was about six feet away the big bird suddenly swung round and pranced forward, long beak thrust out threateningly. The crow in the tree seemed to shout 'Look out', and the other leapt straight in the air with a squawk. He planed round to land ten yards behind the heron again. His opponent now sank his head between his shoulders and appeared to be deep in thought. Emboldened, the crow began a cautious, sidelong approach to within a few yards. Then he tried a new intimidatory tactic. He flew up and down several times with a great commotion of feathers.

The heron took absolutely no notice. When the crow was only a few feet away and stood wagging his head nervously, the heron suddenly straightened his neck and poked his head straight at this tormentor from his full height. This was too much. The ground crow took off defeated and flew to join his pal in the tree from whence we could hear a volley of critical comment proceeding. The heron nonchalantly preened his wing with his beak as if to say, 'I knew he couldn't take it'.

'Come and have a cuppa,' called Elisabeth, who had got a huge thermos flask, plastic cups and chocolate wholemeal biscuits on the brick parapet of the bridge just where the sun shone through a gap in the trees.

'That was better than going to the pictures, Dad,' said Peter, mouth now full of biscuit.

'Yes, all laid on specially for us.'

We drove on looking for a lunch place. It would have to be where we could sit in the car with a nice view, as it really wasn't warm enough to sit out for long. We pulled into the side of a gateway to a field full of South Down sheep. Some were feeding near the gate and the rest were scattered over the field. We took care not to block the gateway, which was just as well, for along came the shepherd with a tractor and trailer. I opened the gate for him and he waved as he drove into the field.

Sheep converged at full tilt from all quarters and stood expectantly around the trailer. The shepherd hauled off a bag of feed and walked along a line of troughs pouring out a regular shower into them as he went. The sheep jostled into place, making two exact lines on either side, with their heads in the trough nibbling up the feed. The shepherd walked back quickly along the line wagging a finger as he passed the sheep.

'A hundred and four,' he muttered at the end.

'How can you be sure you haven't missed one?' asked Peter.

'Practice,' he answered.

Just then, a tweed-clad lady came up on a bicycle with a Bible tucked under her arm. We had seen her turn on to the road from a lane leading down to a church whose tower just thrust above the screen of trees. She looked as if she had just come from teaching at Sunday school.

'Heard a shot in the top wood,' she told the shepherd.

'Thanks. Right, I'll be up there straight away.'

'What's up?' I asked.

'Poachers – there's a load of pheasants in that wood.'

'Will you be able to catch them?'

'Perhaps not, but I'll put the fear of death in 'em.' He laughed and pointed to the tractor cab. I saw the barrels of a twelve-bore shot-gun leaning against the seat. 'Better be off then.'

The tractor chuffed off at a very good pace. Ten minutes later, from the direction of the wood, we heard two loud bangs which sent the rooks wheeling and cawing above the elms. When they had settled, there was a dead silence. Then, from the other side of the wood where the road wound back, we heard a car revving violently. In a minute it came into view roaring down the road towards us, a real old jalopy. It tore by, its occupants huddled and white-faced. I couldn't read the number-plates as they were covered in mud.

'Dad, was that them?' shouted Peter.

'I expect so.' I hadn't recognized any of them. 'You're having an exciting day, Peter!'

'Coo, Dad – just like a western!'

On the way home we were all feeling rather full of lunch and fresh air, and the three children in the back were nearly asleep.

I didn't think that they could have eaten any tea at all after that huge picnic Elisabeth had made – but couldn't they just! After tea, we were all sitting round the fire. Peter got rather quiet. He was always like that about this time. He put off getting his bits and pieces together until the very last moment. Then he was all in a hurry to go.

As we went on the short trip back to the school, Peter turned to me.

'Dad, I like your talk about the rubber glove, but I do

find reading the Bible every morning a bit difficult. I don't really remember anything anyway.'

'Peter, did you hear about the boy whose dad sent him to empty a water butt with a sieve?'

'Don't be silly, Dad. He couldn't.'

'I know, Peter, that's what the boy said, when he came back after trying. His father knew he wouldn't be able to, but he told him to look how clean the sieve was. That's what reading the Bible does for you, even though your head's like a sieve. Bye now, Peter.'

He jumped out, ran across into the doorway. He waved as he stood for a moment in the porch light and then went in.

Next morning, the third patient was a young man I'd never seen before. He limped in and stood by the chair and refused my invitation to sit down. He was a temporary resident staying with his cousins on the housing estate.

'Had an accident with me mates, doc, and got some pellets in me be'ind,' he said.

He had half a dozen shot in his rear end which I spent some time extracting under local anaethestic injections. I didn't ask him where he'd got them – I thought it just as well not to.

16
'Salud'

Elisabeth looked up from *The Wilverton Advertiser*.

'What about taking another look at that house up the farm road? It's still in the "Properties for Sale" section.' She stopped and stared more intently at the paper. 'Andy, I don't believe it! It's been reduced a thousand!'

'Here let me have a look.' I grabbed the newspaper. Sure enough, there it was: £3,800.

I felt an odd thrill. We'd seen the house late the previous

autumn. Buried in a damp copse, it had been badly in need of redecoration. The sitting-room smelt of dogs; the garden was huge and at £4,800 it was outside our range. We'd crossed it off our list but – there had been something about it . . .

We had gone on scanning the adverts. Agents sent us scores of 'desirable properties' we didn't desire. Descriptions revealed great imaginative ability but not the buildings' character. 'Imposing, standing in own spacious grounds' was a Victorian disaster, cheek by jowl with the slaughterhouse. 'Small, individually styled' proved indistinguishable from a largish hen-house.

We became cynical but we didn't lose heart; one day our dream house would come up: not posh, but one with character and room to breathe. After all, our Kenya bungalow had been pretty basic, but the view! There had been a hundred and fifty miles of it!

One day we really thought we'd found it: quiet, old-world, a nicely converted coach-house. Unfortunately or fortunately, I stamped rather hard on a bedroom floor and, next second, my foot was sticking through the dining-room ceiling. As the agent remarked, 'Woodworm is bad in Wilverton'.

But today, today was Saturday, it was May-time and hope was in the air. We'd just go and have another little look, no harm in that. Why the drop in price though? There must be something wrong with the house . . .

We parked the car at the end of the lane and stole down for a private peek. It might have been that £1,000 off, it might have been the spring, but it didn't look the same place. Fruit trees sprinkled with pink and white blossom stood in garlands of daffodils. Bullfinches were adding touches of brilliance as they busily reduced the apple crop. A pair of thrushes were hungrily eyeing the grass and, as we watched, a flock of starlings wheeled in to waddle about in cheeky independence.

Elisabeth drew in her breath. 'Pete's paradise,' she murmured.

'Yours too,' I said. 'You know, we could easily fell one or

two of those trees overhanging the house and put a chunk of the garden at the back down to veg.'

Shafts of sunlight shone through the branches on the half-tiled walls and showed up the patches of orange lichen on the roof. The gable-ends were typical Sussex. In fact, the whole building reminded me of a wholesome loaf of brown bread.

Mrs Parker opened the door to us.

'I'm sorry we haven't an appointment. Do you think we could just see round the house again? You remember, we came before in the autumn.'

She was very nice and let us wander around at will. There was no doubt about it, it was different. No doggy smell, new decorations throughout. From the back bedroom, we looked out on a sea of blossom with the green carpet of the grass showing through the gaps in the trees. Over their tops we could glimpse the Downs.

'Could you tell us what "Salud" means?' I asked Mrs Parker.

'It means "Good health"; the previous owner gave it the name. I must say I've always felt well here myself,' she smiled.

'We would like another look round the garden,' said Elisabeth.

'Certainly.' For a moment Mrs Parker looked sad. 'My husband loved it.'

As we wandered under the fruit trees, Elisabeth whispered, 'I think that's why she's willing to take less – she can't bear the memories.' She paused. ' "Salud" isn't a bad name for a doctor's house – better than Charles's idea of "Bedside Manor" for the house we decide on!'

There was a big cedar hut at the end of the garden.

'What a sun-trap for meals outside.' Elisabeth always rates first what you can do outside a house before the inside.

'What d'you think of the place?' asked Mrs Parker as we went back in. She seemed anxious for us to like it.

It was churlish, but we had been had so many times before, so all I said was, 'Very nice, very nice indeed; we'll be in touch.'

We didn't look at each other as we walked back to the car. I usually have to make the running.

'I think this could be it, 'specially at the price.'

'What about a mortgage?' said Elisabeth.

This was progress! She really seemed on the scent. She continued, 'We've no capital. Can you get a mortgage without capital?'

Neither of us knew. We discussed it all weekend.

On the Tuesday there was one of those coincidences that make you think – or rather two to be precise. In the post was a solicitor's letter telling Elisabeth of a legacy of exactly £550. Number two was when Charles phoned and generously offered a loan of £1,000 at 1 per cent interest.

We rang Mrs Parker's agent and offered the amount she was asking. We were quite green in the matter of house purchasing. We actually thought people asked what they thought the house was worth. The offer was accepted.

Mrs Parker was also rather unsophisticated in the matter of house deals. She wouldn't have known what 'gazumping' was, even if the word had been invented then. The agent told us afterwards that almost immediately she had a much better offer but wouldn't go back on her spoken word to us.

She showed the same lamentable lack of business sense in the rest of her dealings. Everything she sold us only seemed worth £10. The shed £10; a nice Turkey carpet, complete bee-keeping equipment and bees, all £10. The only thing that was different was a motor-mower, that was £5 – oh yes, and the chicken-house, that was free. No chickens, however, but you can't have everything.

She let us come and cultivate the garden before completion. While I dug, the children wandered around in a beatific haze – Peter with his *Observer's Book of Birds*, Sarah visualizing bantams in the hen-house and Barney hissing and whistling round the paths in his role of railway engine.

We'd been grateful for our flat, but only now, as the day of emancipation drew near, did we register the full extent of our tribulations there. An incautious sneeze in the garden could set the neighbourhood curtains fluttering; washing was hung out at night for fear of our being reported to the landlord. Barney had once nearly descended ten feet on to his head when the upstairs verandah rail gave way.

But our sojourn had not been wasted. I had become a familiar figure at auction sales. ' 'E's the one what buys all the junk,' I overheard one day. Very useful junk it proved to be. I developed into a buyer of considerable adroitness and not a little cunning. My one lapse was caused by a cold and the inopportune use of a handkerchief at a crucial point in the proceedings. I inadvertently obtained a seedy-looking divan bed.

When it arrived at the door of the flat, Elisabeth flatly refused it entry. 'Andy, it stinks! Tell the men to take it back.' So it was even as she had said, but we lost £3 on the sale, second time round.

We did not attain the social status of a stair-carpet, not at that time, but I had one notable purchase, using the word 'one' in a generic sense. I arrived late to bid for a ping-pong table at a country-house sale. The auctioneer was holding up a black deed-box. As no one made a bid, I offered two shillings – one shilling seemed a bit niggardly.

'Two shillings I am bid,' said the auctioneer, ill-concealed contempt in his voice. 'Are there any more bids?'

There weren't, so the deed-box was mine and a little later the ping-pong table was too.

Next day, I went to collect my purchases. I found the table.

'Where is Lot 237?' I asked the assistant.

'They're down that passage.'

'They?' I thought. But 'they' it was (or were) – thirty-three of them, deed-boxes in all shapes and sizes, complete with locks and keys. No wonder the auctioneer found my bid unimpressive.

We supplied Charles and Fred with as many as they could be persuaded to take. The rest became tool-boxes, specimen boxes for Peter, medicine boxes, even seed-boxes, but our deeds, when we got some, were kept by the insurance company who lent us the money to buy 'Salud'.

I never had much faith in biblical lucky-dips, especially after hearing the story of the depressed chap who sought guidance by sticking his finger on to a Bible text at random; he got Matthew 27:5, 'He went and hanged himself'. This offered little scope, so he tried again and got Luke 11:37 which told him, 'Go and do thou likewise'. Nevertheless, on the day we moved, our scripture reading set for the day stated, 'The glory of this latter house shall be greater than of the former and in that place will I give peace'.

We didn't feel that the divine prediction for ancient Israel was a talisman for bliss in our new abode, but it was a definite encouragement.

Another was the timely arrival of Joe and Jenny, a young couple *en route* for our part of East Africa. They got into the action with a will. We'd rented a van and we loaded it ourselves under the disapproving windows around. The climax was when Joe staggered forth with a mountainous pile of merchandise. Balanced on the peak was a floral china bedroom receptacle of Barney's. He tripped on the kerb and the crash really set the curtains of the neighbourhood in a twitch.

Joe drove the first load to 'Salud' with Jenny. They had instructions to paint a quick-drying floor-stain on the surrounds of the main bedroom. To this day, when we roll back the carpet for cleaning, we're reminded of their help and humour. Indelibly stained on the centre of the floor are two hearts, pierced by an arrow with the letters 'J.J.' They had, after all, just finished their honeymoon.

We had a week's holiday to cope with the move. Even so, we worked from morn till dusk that first day to create some sort of order and we sank into bed in a state of complete exhaustion. Elisabeth's health had improved wonderfully but when she woke me at about 4 a.m. I was worried in case she had overdone it.

'Andy,' she whispered, and there was no anxiety in her voice, only excitement. 'What d'you think that noise is? Do look out of the window and see.'

I peered cautiously into the dim light of dawn. Below me a beautiful, full-grown badger was standing on his hind legs eating crumbs off the bird-table.

Those early summer days in our new house had a halcyon

quality. Something went wrong with the weather and it was fine for weeks on end. The practice work was unusually slack. Even night-calls lost their strain when you woke afterwards to a dawn chorus of ebbing and flowing bird-song.

'I feel really guilty living here.' I put my cup and saucer down on the grass, my hands behind my head and gazed up. Bunches of tiny apples hung from a branch between me and the scudding clouds. In spite of a breeze, the afternoon sun was warm in the shelter of the open doors of the hut. It was hard to believe we were only five minutes by car from the centre of Wilverton. 'When I think of those terraced houses in the East End of London where I did that job in the war, I wonder why we should have this place to live in.'

'Surely, what matters is being where you ought to be and – being grateful.'

Elisabeth was right – she usually is. She dropped the sock she was darning, picked up the other one and said, 'Shouldn't you be going to surgery?'

I sighed and heaved myself to my feet, 'Bye, love.'

It wouldn't be honest to pretend there weren't snags about 'Salud'. There were. Soon after we got in, the main drain blocked and was dug up and replaced. Then we discovered quite a bit of woodworm in floors and doors which required expensive expert treatment.

The garden had the natural material for years of research into weed and pest control. Ground-elder, couch-grass, bindweed, slugs, caterpillars, canker, pigeons, rabbits and squirrels – you name it, we had it. But nothing dimmed our enjoyment, we still loved the place.

Mother came down with her friend, Mrs Bird, to see us. We set up our second-hand croquet hoops on the grass; they were another minor saleroom triumph, as we aimed to keep the children happy while we sat in the garden. Peter and Sarah, with Denis and Pat from down the road, soon converted a genteel foursome into a pitched battle. At last Mrs Bird could stand it no longer. With the help of her stick, as she was pretty arthritic, she rose from her deck-chair, and advanced on the children.

'Now then,' she said. 'Why don't you play it properly?'

She seized a mallet, made a perfect croquet and then sent the ball ten yards, straight through a hoop.

'Coo, Auntie Bird! How are you so good?' Peter stared in open-eyed admiration.

'Well dear, I did play for England once,' she said mildly.

We gave them asparagus for high tea, cut from the ancient beds at the bottom of the garden.

Word got around about our 'nice house by the sea' and soon 'all rabbit's friends and relations' were queueing to stay. We didn't mind – they all had to do their stint in the garden. Our nearest neighbour unloaded two kittens on us; Pete got a tree-platform to watch birds from, overlooking the pond over the hedge; Sarah soon had her bantams, and Barney had a wigwam under the trees near the house. We could have had a sack of cob-nuts if the squirrels hadn't got there first, but by the time Keats' 'season of mists and mellow fruitfulness' was upon us, our apple trees had produced such a crop that we were reduced to putting boxes of them by the gate for passers-by to take away.

When I felt I'd seen one octogenarian too many, I would seize a spade or a slasher and give that long-suffering garden something to think about. I agree wholeheartedly with Kipling, that,

> The cure for the hump is not to sit still,
> Or froust with a book by the fire;
> But to take a large hoe and a shovel also
> And dig till you gently perspire.

When an old Kenya friend was coming to visit us, we slaved to create a picture of order and cultivation for his benefit. He stood on the back step and looked appreciatively at the scene.

'Beautiful, Andy,' He patted my shoulder. 'Just suits you – semi-wild.'

As leaves began to fall, one night we lay in bed, listening to the wind in the trees and the hoot of an owl close by.

I held Elisabeth's hand in the darkness.

'I *am* grateful darling, truly grateful.'

There was no denying it: 'Salud' was just what the doctor ordered.

17

Discernment

'You've only yourself to blame,' Charles spoke with bland authority. 'It's all a matter of discernment – an essential quality. I'm not suggesting you become a suspicious type, but, having got all the facts, taking nothing on trust, come to a decision and there you are. Never fails, discernment.'

I resisted the temptation to deflate him by telling him about the patient I'd seen that morning, a Mrs Bryson. She's a sweet old octogenarian and she was very upset.

'Dr Hamilton, I've come specially to see you. You must tell me what Dr Semple meant when I saw him last night.'

'Why, what did he say?'

'He said I had a chronic complaint with no cure, which would be fatal in the end.'

'Did he give it a name?'

'He said I was suffering from Annie Dominie.'

I relieved her fears, but I felt that Charles's discernment ought to take account of the patient's reaction to his dry humour as well. Still, I had to admit he'd got a point. I was the one who'd been taken in the week before.

She was so small and woebegone as she sat by my desk. She was twenty-five but looked a good bit older.

'Can you tell me what's wrong, Mrs Whitford?'

'It's this pain here,' and she put her hand over her left breast. 'It comes and goes – sort of aches.'

'When do you get it?'

'When I'm sitting in the evening. Goes off when I'm around during the day.'

It didn't sound cardiac, more nervous in origin, or a sub-conscious desire to get a ticket to see the doctor.

'How are you sleeping?'

'Now that's the trouble, doctor. I can't. Oh doctor, it's my husband.' It came out with a rush. 'I think he hates me. Keeps waking me up all night long.'

It sounded bad, and they'd only been married ten months. It looked as if the marriage was already breaking up. I made sure that her heart and chest were really sound, and then I tried to sort things out, but I'm afraid not very successfully.

Then I had a brainwave. This was just the sort of situation for Algernon.

'Would you mind if I asked Mr Greenfield to call on you and have a talk? He might be able to help you.'

She seemed rather pleased with the suggestion. So I rang him up and gave him a run-down on her case and he said he'd try to help.

I heard from him two days later.

'How did you get on, Algie?'

'I agree the marriage is slipping,' he replied. 'But if Mrs Whitford didn't smoke in bed it would make things a lot easier. She falls asleep with lighted cigarettes in her mouth and she's twice burnt holes in the blankets. Her husband is dead scared she'll set the place on fire so he wakes her up.'

It was a good thing this conversation was on the telephone. He couldn't see my face. I felt a right charlie – especially as I remembered her yellowed fingers and smoker's breath.

'I'm sorry Algie, but I'm grateful for your help.'

'Discernment', Charles had said!

Even without possessing much of it, I was put off Robinson from the start. Anybody who tries to bully our good Miss Spencer is on a sticky wicket with me straightaway.

He was a 'foreigner' from London, and he'd bought the run-down garage in Albemarle Street – one of the mews roads behind the main street, running down to the front.

We don't accept applications to join the practice over the telephone. We reckon that patients and practice have the right to see one another before becoming involved with each other. Robinson had other ideas and he let Miss Spencer know in no uncertain terms. She doesn't often do it, but this time she asked if I'd take over. I held the phone about three inches from my ear as a powerful blast of cockney came over.

'What's all this fiddle-faddle abaht? Me last doctor didn't want a personal inspection before 'e took us on. Diabolical liberty, I calls it.'

There was a lot more like that. I waited until he ran out of steam before answering.

'You can call it what you like, Mr Robinson,' I was all sweet reasonableness. 'But we find it works best for both parties this way, so you can take it or leave it. No one's compelling you to come on our list.'

His swallowing was audible. I imagined he was used to swamping opposition and wasn't prepared for straight talking.

'Oh, all right. I'll get the missus to bring the cards round.'

'Thank you, Mr Robinson, then we'll be able to come to a decision as to whether you should become our patients. Goodbye.'

Mrs Robinson brought them round next day, and asked straightaway if we could see her. It was the first of many visits. Robinson himself we never saw professionally. 'Bert's never ill,' she told me.

She could have been a nice-looking woman with her big blue eyes and slightly turned-up nose, but she'd spoilt the effect by bleaching her hair and overdoing the styling. A chocolate-box appearance didn't mask her scared look. She had a wide variety of complaints: headache, breathlessness, attacks of vertigo, pains in the chest, loss of appetite and sleeplessness. After examination and tests, this unrelated collection of symptoms only indicated one thing: psychosomatic illness. She confessed at last to unreasoning fears.

'Are you and your husband in trouble? Have you a good relationship? Have you financial worries?'

She shook her head to all my questions.

'Money's not the trouble, doctor. He don't keep me short, but things ain't the same as they was in London. 'E never seems to 'ave no time for anything, not for me or the 'ouse. You see, we never 'ad no kids – something about me ovaries, the specialist said. Sex don't worry me, and Bert seems to have lost interest in that sort of thing. Wish we were back in the Old Kent Road with our breaker's yard. We was 'appy then even though we 'adn't two brass farthings to rub together. It's ever since Bert started doing better, 'e changed. I'm scared doctor, I'm scared. Specially when 'e's going on them Continental trips, buying them cars. No, I don't think 'e 'as another woman on the side, but 'e's so short, won't 'ardly speak after them trips. I can't sleep for worryin'. That's what me old doctor gave me them sleeping capsules for. Seconal they were called. I must 'ave 'em, doctor. Don't sleep a wink without. You will give me some, won't you?'

'Well, I'll give you a small supply, Mrs Robinson, but we must see if we can sort out your worries and get you off them soon.'

I gave her a prescription for twenty-five one and a half grain capsules, 'one to be taken at night'.

I wondered about Bert. Was he on the fiddle? Car-breaking and then selling new and second-hand cars – stolen perhaps, some of them? It would explain his irritability, but was it my affair? Well, if I were to help his wife, I needed to know whether she had cause for her fears or if they were only imagination.

A business contact with him didn't do anything to allay my suspicions, and yet it was only something a lot of dealers take as a matter of course. It paid to exchange cars frequently, because you got a good price for the old one, and you got no major repair bills. The only snag was tax allowance on depreciation. If you got too much for the old car, it was more than the written-down value and it reduced the tax allowance.

Although I felt unpatriotic, I felt I'd like to try a Volkswagen 'Beetle' as I knew they were very reliable. Bert imported these as well as French cars. This was why he made trips to the Continent to negotiate the purchase. He made me a good offer for my old car, even though the differential had started to whine.

'Pity I'll lose on tax rebate,' I remarked ruefully.

'Don't let that worry you, doc.' Bert smirked and shifted his cigar to the other side of his mouth. 'No skin off my nose. I've got a buyer for your old bus all lined up. What if I knock off £100 on the exchange value of your bus, give you £100 in cash and no one's any the wiser. What d'yer say?'

I tried not to sound too priggish. After all, though it was dishonest, he was trying to do me a favour.

'Sorry, Mr Robinson. We'll let the original deal stand, shall we?'

He flushed. 'OK, guv. Whatever you say. It's your money.'

I loved that little bus. It handled like a racing car after the Vauxhall I had been driving, but I noticed a pull to the left when I was braking, so at the first service I asked for this to be put right. I hadn't driven it far before I could feel it was just as bad after the service as before. I went back and had some words with Robinson. He got out the charge sheet. There it was: 'Adjust brakes'. He opened the office window on to the workshop.

'George,' he shouted. In came the older mechanic. 'Who did that job on the doctor's car?' Robinson asked.

'It was Bob Hansford,' said George.

'Send 'im in.'

Bob looked sheepish. I noticed his hands were shaking.

'Did you adjust the doctor's brakes?'

'Sorry boss, I forgot,' he answered.

'Now look 'ere.' It was that bullying tone I'd heard on the phone. 'If you can't do a job you're asked to, you're no good to me. Watch it, or you'll get your cards. Right? Now go and do them brakes.'

I was sorry for the lad. He'd a strange look and I didn't like those trembling hands, but I probably would have forgotten all about it if Mrs Hansford hadn't turned up at the surgery a week later. She was in a terrible state.

'I'm sorry, doctor. I haven't come for myself. It's Robert. He's not right. Terribly moody, sometimes all excited, then he's real sulky. Bites my head off if I speak a word out of place. He didn't eat his food properly today either. That boy's not well. I know him. He's been going downhill for months. Different boy from what he used to be. I had to come – he won't come himself.'

Poor Mrs Hansford. Her husband had been a tail gunner in the raids on Germany and he'd been shot down in 1944 when Robert was a baby.

'Misses having a dad. Isn't sure of himself, no real self-confidence, doctor, but he got four O-levels at school, Maths,

Physics, Chemistry and English, though he was in a state before the exams.'

'I'll come round one evening and have a chat, Mrs Hansford.'

'Oh thank you, doctor. I'd be so grateful.'

What was it Charles had said? 'You don't have to be suspicious. Get all the facts, take nothing on trust . . . discernment.' I needed discernment now. I felt I hadn't all the facts but I was certainly getting suspicious. No self-confidence, change of mood, forgetting his duties and those trembling hands . . . but before I got around to visiting Robert Hansford, his mother was back.

Miss Spencer pushed her into the evening surgery out of turn by telling her to wait outside my door and ringing me on the internal phone, to ask me to let her in before I buzzed for the next patient.

'He's gone, doctor.'

'What do you mean "gone"?'

'He's left home. Packed some things and left. Hasn't gone to work today either. I telephoned Mr Robinson and made some excuse when he wanted to know where Bob was.'

'Now you go home, Mrs Hansford, and I'll see if I can find him.'

She calmed down at last and left.

As soon as surgery was over, I rang the police station and asked for Sergeant Jones. Fortunately he was still on duty.

'Dai, do you know of any hide-outs where yobbos go, in or around the town somewhere? It might be a question of drugs. I'm looking for a lad called Bob Hansford.'

'Well, doctor, there's a disused farm cottage belonging to the Thornbarrow estate on the edge of town. It's up a track behind a chestnut plantation. Woodcutters slept in it about ten years ago when they last cut the woods. I believe some youngsters have used it as a hang-out.'

'Thanks, Dai. I'll be seeing you.'

I stopped my car at the edge of the woodland and walked the last hundred yards. It was a little hip-roofed Sussex cottage which could have been made quite charming if the undergrowth had been cleared and the whole place cleaned up and repainted. A trickle of grey smoke was coming from the chimney. I knocked on the door. I knocked again and stood back.

A half-dressed, tousle-haired youth put his head out of a first-floor window about two feet above the porch.

'What d'you want?' he said, without any marked show of friendliness.

'Is Bob Hansford here? I'm his doctor.'

The head was withdrawn. I listened.

'Here Bob, there's a quack wanting you.'

About three minutes later, Bob opened the door about a foot.

'Hullo, doctor. What can we do for you?' He was bleary-eyed and euphoric.

'Look here, Bob,' I whispered. 'You're worrying the life out of your mum, and I want you to come back with me now. I know you're on drugs.'

'Sorry doc, nothing doing.'

He lifted his bare arm in a ludicrous wave and I saw the puncture-marks on the front surface of his elbow. Then he shut the door in my face.

I called on Mrs Hansford on my way home with a feeling of utter failure. It wasn't helped by the sight of her ashen face when I told her he wouldn't come home. The worst was yet to come. Two days later, Sergeant Dai Jones rang me up in the afternoon.

'Doc, you know that lad you asked me about the other day, name of Hansford? I'm sorry to tell you he was picked up for shop-lifting this afternoon, the young fool. Must be crazy, it was so obvious. The shop detective saw him in action. I wondered if you wanted to do anything to help him. We've charged him.'

'Thanks for letting me know, Dai.'

Two days later it was a shaken, pallid young man that I found when I called. He was coming up for trial in Brighton and he was scared. When he was arrested it had been 'cold turkey' for him in the cell, that awful experience of sudden deprivation of hard drugs. He was over that now and his mother, bless her, had swallowed her fears now she knew the worst, and was acting with a restraint and understanding I hadn't thought her capable of. She went to the kitchen to make some tea and Bob came clean.

'It all started, doctor, when I was at school. I was scared of people, scared of exams, scared of life. I had just one pal and when he said "Why don't you try some of these, give you some guts it will", I thought I would. It was purple hearts. I didn't want to really but I couldn't face the exams, so I tried a couple. I went into those exams as if I couldn't care less. That was the start.

'Later on we began going over to Brighton on his motor bike and met some other guys who smoked reefers. Then one of 'em got some snow and like fools we tried it. Doctor, we've had it. We only used it on and off at first but then I found an easy way to get it, and I started mainlining.'

'How did you manage to get it?'

'Doctor, I can't tell you.'

'Now look here Bob, you're in a jam. For one thing, if you know a pusher and help the police it will help you, and for another, what about the other poor guys whose lives he's ruining? Don't you want to help them?'

'I'm sorry, doctor, I can't tell you. You don't understand, I just daren't.'

I couldn't budge him. I don't know about discernment, but I was getting mighty suspicious again. Facts were falling into place and they were all pointing one way. But I'd got no concrete evidence.

Before I could do anything about it events got out of hand. In general practice, you're pretty tied up. People aren't ill to order and the daily work had to be done.

Bob Hansford came up for trial. I had told the solicitor who was acting for Bob under legal aid that I would speak for him. I was prepared to testify to Bob's general character and undertake to arrange for him to be admitted to an institution to get him off drugs.

I knew of a place in the Midlands which took young men who'd got hooked and wanted to get off; they had to have them referred to them from the courts under probation and this was accepted sometimes as an alternative to a prison sentence. The institution was run by a Christian group. There was strong discipline and their record for permanent cures was better than anywhere else in the world.

Bob's plea was that he was under drugs, and therefore not fully responsible for his actions in shop-lifting, to which he admitted. He was given a conditional discharge provided he came under my care to help him get rid of the drug habit. I saw Bob off with the probation officer from the station, and heaved a sigh of relief.

Then the real tragedy happened.

It was a neighbour ringing.

'Doctor, come at once please. I can't get any reply from Mrs Robinson. I'm sure she's in. Maybe she's been taken ill, and can't come to the door.'

Immediately it flashed into my mind. 'She's taken an overdose, I must get there at once.'

'Elisabeth, call the ambulance, darling, and send them to the Robinsons'. They live in the main road, number eighty-three, in front of their garage in Albemarle Mews.'

In a matter of minutes I was there. I rang the bell, tried the front door – but it was useless. There was no reply and I couldn't get in. I went down the side passage at the back facing on to the mews and tried the back door. It was locked too.

Then I smelt it. Coal gas, unmistakable! I drew back and threw all my weight on the door. The lock burst off and the door flew in. Mrs Robinson was lying with her head in the gas oven. Holding my breath, I grabbed her and dragged her out, then whipped back and turned off the taps.

She was quite dead – cold, stiff and blue. She must have been dead for some hours. Then my mind started to race – she was *blue*! She should have been *pink* if she'd died from gas poisoning. Her blood vessels would have contained a great deal of carboxy-haemoglobin if she'd died from the carbon monoxide in coal gas, and blood like that is pink, not the dark bluish colour of blood with haemoglobin deprived of oxygen.

One thing was certain, she had been dead before she was put in the gas oven! But who had put her there, and how had she died? I began to feel that I could make a pretty good guess.

The ambulance men arrived and I told them they needn't wait, the patient was dead, it was a coroner's job and I would have to get the police to arrange transport to the mortuary. I walked through the yard, out of the back gate and over the mews road into the garage.

'Where's the boss?' I asked, though I thought I knew the answer they would give.

'He's over in France, guv, buying Peugeots,' said the head mechanic.

'Can I use the office phone please? It's urgent.'

'What's up, guv?'

'Mrs Robinson. I'm afraid she's dead.'

'No! Cor, and the boss away! In 'ere, doc.'

The woman police constable at the switchboard answered. 'Can I help you?'

'Dr Hamilton. Give me the CID please.'

'CID. What can I do for you?'

'Dr Hamilton. I have a death, in suspicious circumstances. Mrs Robinson, 83 Main Road.'

'We'll be with you straightaway, doctor.'

It was Sergeant Dai Jones and another plain-clothes detective who came.

'Found her with her head in the gas oven,' I said, as Dai lifted off poor Mrs Robinson's face the coat I'd thrown over her.

'Suicide?' he said.

'No, could be murder.'

He raised his eyebrows.

'How come, doc?'

'She's the wrong colour. She should be pink. Look at her.'

He looked.

'I know you'll go over the place with a tooth-comb, but I would particularly like to see where she was in bed.'

'OK, doc. I'll lead the way, but don't touch anything until I say, will you?'

The bed looked just as if it had been slept in. There were no signs of a struggle. The bottle of seconal was in a drawer.

135

I always instructed patients to put their drugs away and not to keep them by the bedside table in case they accidentally overdosed themselves in a half-doped state. I did a quick calculation from the remaining two or three capsules. Unless she had saved them up for the occasion, Mrs Robinson hadn't taken an overdose.

'May I look at the pillows?' I asked Sergeant Jones.

'OK.'

I lifted them. The cases looked virtually unused.

'Excuse me.' I went into the bathroom.

There was quite a lot of soiled linen in a dirty clothes-basket. I called Dai. He took the things out one by one and, half-way down, he found what I was looking for: a pillow-slip, and in the middle on one side a patch still damp showing faint blood smears and a ragged tear that could have been done by teeth.

I showed Dai.

'Can we have another quick look at the body?' I asked him.

We had lifted her back into the kitchen; the gas had cleared now. There were faint diffuse bruises on the forearm under the long sleeves of her nightdress.

'Dai, I'm going to write a report. I think Mrs Robinson was suffocated when asleep on a dose of seconal and her body dumped in the gas stove to make it look like suicide. If I'm right, I have to suppose a murderer wouldn't know about her being the wrong colour.'

'Got anybody in mind, doc?'

I hesitated – after all, Robinson was my patient too. But I decided I owed more loyalty to the dead than the living.

''Fraid so, Dai; Mr Robinson.'

'Eh?' Dai's eyebrows rose again. 'Why him?'

'Well, it's a long shot. I can't prove it, Dai.'

'Try me.' Dai's eyes had a professional if slightly in-credulous gleam.

'You know that lad Hansford, who was on drugs. He worked for Robinson, as you know, and he was getting easy supplies of heroin from somewhere. Robinson seems to be doing uncommonly well financially even though he's only got

136

a small show here, and his wife was worried stiff about him, especially when he went on the Continent to buy cars.

'Now, suppose he was smuggling drugs on his return trips and suppose somehow young Hansford found out. There could have been a lot of mutual pressure going on. Robinson supplying Hansford in return for silence, and Hansford depending on Robinson for supplies. If I'm right, it was a dangerous situation for both but perhaps there was no alternative at the start.

'It's a lot of supposes, but what if Mrs Robinson found out too about his drug-smuggling and made him promise to pack it in and he promised he would go across to the Continent and wind it up but instead sneaked back at night, let himself in, knowing she was on sleeping capsules and put that pillow on her face and then really went over to France today?'

Dai's face was a study. 'If you're right, you've missed your vocation, doc. Should have been a forensic specialist.'

'No, Dai,' I said miserably. 'It's just my suspicious nature, but I'm too late.' I looked down at the shape on the floor.

I got the full story afterwards. Dai spent the morning on the phone, working through the Channel ports and at last he got the information he wanted. Yes, a Mr Robinson had travelled on the first boat to Boulogne from Folkestone that morning with his car.

What a mad risk he'd taken. A message went through to Interpol to pick him up for questioning. But they couldn't stop the evening papers getting the story that Mrs Robinson had been murdered, and the French papers apparently picked it up.

Robinson was found in his car, down a quiet lane near Boulogne, with a tube from the exhaust through the window. When they took the car to pieces, they found a neat little compartment in the structure of the front seat and there were traces of heroin still in it. With macabre poetic justice, the French post-mortem report stated, *'La peau c'est rose'*.

It was nine months later that young Robert Hansford came in to see me. He looked sunburnt and fit.

'Thanks for getting me to that centre, doc. I'm off drugs

for good, and better still, I'm a real Christian now and I know where I can find strength just to accept myself as I am and do something for other people into the bargain.'

18

A tale of two sisters

The girl was pretty and knew how to dress, but the shadows under her eyes and the pallor of her cheeks made me cut out my usual cheerful greetings.

I glanced up again from the record-card on my pad.

'What can I do for you, Miss Evans?'

She hesitated. 'I'm not really sure, doctor. I don't know how to put it – I just don't feel well. I've been off my food for three weeks now, the mere sight of it turns my stomach – specially first thing in the morning.'

A thought – not a particularly subtle one – was simmering in my head. I wasn't going to jump to conclusions however.

'What is your work?'

'I'm a ward sister at the Duke of Gloucester.'

Well, I thought, it could be strain. Long hours, difficult patients, staff problems – yes – it could lead to anorexia. Yet somehow I didn't believe it. Ward sisters like this girl were usually made of sterner stuff.

I wanted to avoid asking an embarrassing question that could be quite wide of the mark so I went on obliquely, working through the bodily functions, waiting for a lead.

'Have you any abdominal pain? Do you suffer with headaches? Any trouble with the waterworks or bowels – how about your periods?'

At this last question, she stopped shaking her head and her pale face flushed.

'I haven't seen anything for three months, doctor.'

It was natural to follow this up.

'Have you felt any discomfort in the breasts?'

'Yes, doctor.'

I got up and opened the door to the examination-room.

'Will you go in there and undress sufficiently for me to examine your tummy?'

I rang for Miss Spencer and sent her in with Miss Evans.

'All ready, doctor,' she called.

Sure enough, I could feel the uterus, two fingers' breadth above the pubic synphysis.

'Thank you, Miss Spencer. That's all.'

When Sister Evans came back and sat down, I told her, 'There's very little doubt about it. I should think you are about fourteen weeks' pregnant.'

Her eyes had that odd mixture of fear and triumph that women show, even when a pregnancy is unintended. Maybe their full womanhood is being proclaimed to themselves and to the world at large.

As she sat there, her left hand lying on the desk, I could see she was trembling. For the first time, I noticed her engagement ring.

'Are you planning to get married soon?'

Her eyes filled with tears.

'My fiancé was killed two months ago in a motor cycle accident.'

Instinctively I put out my hand to hers.

'I'm very sorry, I had no idea; but, now you've told me, I remember seeing about the accident in the local paper.'

When she regained her composure, I released her hand.

'I'd better write to the consultant as this is your first pregnancy.' (I felt sure it was, even without asking.) 'You should be under hospital care.'

'Oh, I couldn't do that, doctor. Not in my own hospital!'

I saw I'd been a bit insensitive. I should have thought of her feelings more.

The abortion law was as yet unchanged and the agonizing choice of whether to allow a pregnancy to continue or not was rarely faced by a woman or her doctor, except when the mother's life or health was in serious danger. In any event, I felt certain that terminating her pregnancy had not even entered her head. Her baby was the fruit of a genuine if untimely union, and she wanted it – wanted it badly, without a shadow of doubt.

The pill, with its benefits and its invitation to casual sex, was just becoming available, but this girl was the sort who would normally have regarded sexual relations as an integral part of the total commitment of marriage. A moment of passion – not forgetting to take her pill – had put her in her present position, and she wasn't looking for an easy way out. She only wanted to avoid notice.

'Doctor, let me have a talk with my parents and see what we can arrange before you do anything – please.'

'Of course – just as you say – but I'll help you all I can.'

A week later, she was back. Her face was ashen.

'My mother and father don't want to know. They say I've disgraced the family and I'd better go and have the baby quietly somewhere else. They say they can't be involved.'

I barely managed to stop myself saying what I felt about this self-protective and self-righteous inhumanity.

'Don't worry. I know a society in Croydon who will put you up for the latter part of your pregnancy, they'll arrange for your delivery in the local maternity unit and give you post-natal care until you can manage on your own. Could you get a room in the nurses' home here for a few weeks? I'll do your antenatals for the time being.'

'Oh doctor, I would be so grateful. When I left my parents, I just didn't know what I was going to do.' Her face brightened and the despair in her eyes died away.

I was glad her parents weren't patients of mine. Our relations would have become somewhat strained.

The secretary to the society sent a kind letter of acceptance. Two weeks later Sister Evans offered her resignation, and, after working out her month's notice, left with my letter for the doctor attending the maternity home, giving her history to date. As she would be leaving my list, her record would be transferred to him, but the wheels of the Health Service would grind too slowly for them to reach him in time to be much help in her early care.

So Sister Evans faded out of my life.

Practice work went on – the routine highlighted by the occasional medical triumph, but more often than not simply by the feeling that someone had been helped to go through the tunnel of fear or suffering and to emerge in the daylight, all the brighter for the dark left behind.

'Put yourself in the patient's place, that's what you've got to attempt,' Charles would say. 'What matters is to give the last patient the same time and attention as the first – after all, he's waited longer to get it!'

Mrs Frances' visit was last, but it was certainly not her first! We'd looked after her for years – mostly with her numerous babies. She was what's known technically as a 'grande multip' and here she was, pregnant again. Bringing up her family hadn't been easy on her husband's pay as a shop assistant in one of Wilverton's old-established ladies' millinery and dress shops. But she'd kept them together and, barring the usual rows when teenagers scent freedom and parents danger, they were a united bunch. She'd been a sister at the Duke of Gloucester, but left when her first baby was on the way.

'This is where we came in,' I said breezily, but Mrs Frances was not feeling breezy. She didn't beat about the bush either.

'Doctor, I can't go through with this pregnancy. I want an abortion.'

The new Act of Parliament was now in force and, according to its broad intent, there were grounds for termination if it could be held that continuation of the pregnancy was detrimental to the well-being of the existing family. Not that I agreed with the concept as it stood. Along with many other doctors, I felt that it opened the way to abortion on demand and disregarded the unborn child's right to live.

But, this wasn't the time to launch into a dissertation on my personal convictions. Here was a strong woman in deep distress and I had other convictions about her.

'Mrs Frances,' I spoke very gently. 'This baby has started very late in your life. I realize that. But, you're fit. Why are you really asking for an abortion? What's the real reason? I know you love babies!'

It was a fact established beyond dispute. She was at her best with her children. Not only that, given half the chance, she would fill the remaining space in her home with the neighbours' offspring as well, and revel in it. Her elder daughter too was a chip off the old block – couldn't be happy unless she was looking after the local kids.

Nature had designed Mrs Frances as a Grade A Mum. What had brought her to the point of asking for an abortion? It was quite out of character.

For a full moment she stared at the floor. I could see she was wrestling with herself. Then she looked me straight in the eye.

'It's no good trying to fool you, doctor. I want this baby. I want it as much as any of my other kids but – look at our home! What sort of a place is that for a baby? It's cramped, it's dilapidated. It's got three bedrooms and one living-room. You know what it's like. You can't have six people cooped up in there without it getting knocked about. We haven't a hope of a transfer unless we can get it done up, and how are we going to do that on my husband's pay?'

I pictured the house: clean – yes, as clean as an ex-hospital sister could keep it, but with doors needing paint, handles loose, ceilings dark and peeling, wallpaper tatty and faded. Just what you'd expect from too many people and too little money.

'Is that really the only reason why you want an abortion?' She nodded.

'Look, will you get the family together one evening next week? Not Monday, I'll be half-dead after surgery. I'd like to have a word with them. Do they know about the baby?' She shook her head. 'Well, may I tell them?'

She nodded again, her eyes examining me curiously.

'Tuesday?' she asked.

'Right, I'll be there. About eight. Make sure all the family's in, especially Cedric.'

That was her husband. Bit tough being called Cedric – the only other one I know is Little Lord Fauntleroy. It sort of type-casts you, a name like Cedric.

When I walked in they were all there, even the eldest,

who'd got off night school for the occasion. There wasn't much room in the fifteen by twelve living-room. They were sitting around, awkwardly, on the edges of their chairs, distinctly apprehensive.

'Nice, seeing you all in one piece, instead of having something needing mending,' I started. 'Don't look so worried, you haven't done anything – it's what I hope you're going to do that I've come about.'

I took a deep breath.

'Mum is going to have another baby.'

If I'd hoped for a round of applause I was disappointed; only the elder girl's eyes lit up. It was a non-event as far as the others were concerned.

'But', I went on, 'this house is too small to fit another baby into – and you won't get a transfer to a bigger one unless this is in a good deal better condition than it is now. That's right, isn't it, Mr Frances?'

'You're right, doctor.' His tone was hardly inspirational. He sucked his pipe. He was a good chap but lacking initiative, except in the matter of increasing the population.

He took his pipe out.

'Cost a fortune, it would, to set it to rights.'

'I agree. But, suppose you did it yourselves – cost only the materials then!'

He still looked doubtful. It was a bit underhand, but I could see I'd got to pressurize him a bit.

'What about it you lot? Are you on – all help Dad?'

'Come on, Dad – let's have a bash. We can do it!' Geoffrey, the one at night school, looked cheerfully at his dad. 'I could chip in a bit out of me wages to help.'

Before Cedric could reply, his wife, who had slipped out during the discussion, came in with mugs of tea on a tray and they all started talking at once. Dad fished out an inch tape, designed for measuring dress-lengths, and started calculating the wall area. I was forgotten. I swigged my tea and moved quietly to the door.

Mrs Frances followed. 'Thanks, doctor. They'll do it – I know they will.'

When I had to call four weeks later to see Tommy, the

six-year-old, who had tonsillitis, I hardly recognized the place.

Mrs Frances was justly proud of the achievement. Maybe orange floral paper combined with bright pink skirting-boards and door isn't everyone's cup of tea, but the general effect was impressive. And it impressed the housing inspector to the extent of allocating a four-bedroom, two living-room house a few streets away, to the Frances family.

Mrs Frances produced her fifth baby with a skill born of long practice. The family absorbed little Jacqueline, and, with the extra rooms, the squash was only as bad as it had been before her arrival.

Around the time that Mrs Frances had her final post-natal, I was waiting one morning in the surgery for the next patient to come in. The temporary resident form read 'Mrs Dalton'. The name meant nothing to me, but I sat up with a jerk when she came in.

'Sister Evans' stood there smiling. She had matured, become almost matronly (in an unprofessional sense), but she was as charming as ever – and obviously 'expecting'! By her side was a thirteen-year-old, a small edition of herself.

'Well, Mrs Dalton, what can we do for you?'

'I don't need anything, doctor; perhaps I shouldn't be using up surgery time, but I'm down seeing Mum and Dad and I did want to see you and bring May. She has a new daddy and a brother and a sister – and', she blushed, 'another on the way.

'We're a very happy family. The people at the society in Croydon you sent me to were so good and kind when May was coming. I felt quite at home there, and I found a real faith through what they did for me. I just wanted to thank you.'

She held out her hand and I shook it and then May's, and out they went.

Thoughtfully I tore up the temporary resident card and dropped the bits in the waste-paper basket. I couldn't claim a fee for that interview! I'd been well rewarded anyhow.

I caught a glimpse of my face in the mirror as I sat down: it bore an inane grin. Why had I felt so jaded? Why had the view from the surgery window seemed so bleak? It was a *lovely* day – full of interest and opportunity. Would I swap jobs with anyone? Not a chance! I positively punched the bell for the next patient.

The story of the Frances baby had a bitter-sweet finale.

Instead of being a discarded foetus in a hospital bucket, Jacqueline was a sturdy infant, crowing and crying, keeping her mother (and her eldest sister) fully occupied. Soon she was filling a space in their lives – one that suddenly became desperately empty.

When Jacqueline was three months old, Tommy was running home from school with his friends and suddenly, for no apparent reason, he ran across the road in the path of a car.

He died on the way to hospital.

19

Buttercup Joe

Surgery was over and Fred and I were busy sharing out the visits in the day-book. Suddenly the date at the top reminded me – hardly any shopping days to Christmas, and I was in my usual state of unreadiness. I put my pen down and gave vent to my thoughts, which were now nothing to do with the cases in the book.

'I'd love to get a decent radio for Elisabeth – she dearly likes classical music and the reproduction on our present little set is terrible.'

'You should get her a good speaker,' said Fred. 'That would help a lot.'

'I doubt if I could afford it, I expect they cost the earth.'

'Why don't you go and see if Joe Butterworth could help you? He's got loads of old sets. He'd sell you a second-hand speaker for next to nothing – that is, if you don't mind it not being too posh.'

'I couldn't care less so long as the tone's good. Who's Joe Butterworth?'

'I thought you would know him – he's a local character. Lives in Aberdeen Row in the old town. I got a nice radio-gram from him a year or so ago – nothing to look at, but good quality sound. There's only one trouble about Joe, and that's paying him! He just never sends a bill in.'

'Sounds like a man after my own heart!' I grinned.

Everyone was trying to get their ailments cured before Christmas so there wasn't much free time for me to see Mr Butterworth, but at last I had a call to make in his part of the town. After I'd seen the patient, I went on to find his house. It wasn't difficult. The garden of the terraced cottage was full of broken-down old radios, rolls of wire and – curiouser and curiouser – several bulging sacks with very strong-smelling contents.

I banged the door-knocker. It echoed loudly through the house, but no one came. I tried again, but still there was no response. Then I saw a side passage leading round the back.

I followed it down and found myself in a long back garden with a shed near the bottom. Beyond it was a chicken-run and more sacks. I walked down to the shed, the atmosphere becoming vaguely reminiscent of a rubbish-tip. From inside came a continuous grinding noise, rather like a rusty mowing machine. Wires sagged precariously from the back of the house to the shed. I hammered on the door.

The noise came to a stop, the door opened and a grey-haired man of about fifty looked out. His face was quiet and kindly but it was curiously grey and flabby, with pouches under the eyes. He smiled and opened the door. His clothes were baggy and he stooped.

'What can I do for you?' he asked. His voice was unexpectedly deep and hoarse.

'Doctor Wilson sent me. He thought you might have an old speaker you could sell me, to improve the reproduction from my wireless. I'd like a ten-inch one, if you have such a thing?'

'Well, I might have,' he answered. 'Shall we go and have a look?'

He turned back to his machinery and clicked a switch. The apparatus consisted of a battered electric motor connected by a belt to an ancient sausage-meat machine. Several more sacks lay open on the floor. He was grinding up stale bread and scraps, I presumed to feed to his chickens.

He led the way back into the house. As we went in, I could hardly believe my eyes. Apart from the kitchen and a small area around the fireplace in the dining-room, the whole ground floor was stacked with wirelesses in various stages of disrepair, and with other radio equipment. He poked around, shook his head and beckoned me to follow him upstairs.

The scene there was similar. There weren't any sets actually in the bath or on his bed, but they lay in heaps everywhere else. Batteries, valves and reels of electric cable filled up odd corners.

'How about this?' He spoke again in that curious hoarse voice. I noted that although the house was quite warm, he hadn't taken off his old overcoat. My medical nose began to twitch. He pulled out an old walnut-veneered cabinet. It had a ten-inch speaker with a faded silk screen behind fretwork.

'That would be fine,' I answered. 'How much is it?'

He hesitated. 'I'll have to think about it.'

I remembered Fred's warning.

'Now, Mr Butterworth. I must pay you for it before I take it away.'

He sighed.

'Well . . . thirty shillings then,' he said at last, as if taking money gave him a pain.

As I gave it to him, my hand touched his for a second. His skin was very cold.

He insisted on trying out the speaker before I took it away. We lugged it downstairs and he connected it to a small set in the living-room. Maybe it wasn't up to a modern music centre job, but it sounded good to me – especially with the bass notes booming out satisfactorily.

I looked at Mr Butterworth again.

'Will you excuse me,' I said, 'but I'm a doctor myself and I can't help noticing your voice. Has it always been hoarse?'

He looked shyly at me out of the corner of his eye.

'No,' he grated.

'Have you seen a doctor?'

He seemed to wilt a little.

'Don't go in for them myself,' he said. 'No offence, of course.'

'Would you mind if I felt your pulse?' I asked, and took his wrist before he could back away. The rate was about fifty. 'How have you been recently?' I persisted.

'Fair enough.'

'Do you feel the cold badly?' I indicated his overcoat.

'Curious you should ask – I'm freezing even on a warm day. My lady-friend has been telling me to get an iron tonic for a long time.'

Somehow I couldn't picture him with a lady-friend, but I said, 'Look, you need more than a tonic. I think you're suffering from an under-acting thyroid gland – myxoedema, the condition's called. The bellows of the body's fire aren't blowing and you're cooling down. I think a simple treatment with thyroid tablets would set you right, but you'd need them daily and probably for an indefinite period.'

To my surprise he didn't need further cajoling.

'Could you give them to me?' he asked.

'Yes, but you'd have to register with our practice unless you want to pay for them – then you'd have to pay me too!' I smiled. 'No need for that – that's what the Health Service is for. I've got a card in the car you can sign. Of course, you're free to apply to any doctor you like – you don't have to come to me.'

He grinned. 'I think I'll have you, please.'

I went to the car and fetched the card and my prescription pad. Mr Butterworth had disappeared, so I wrote out a prescription: 'Thyroid gn I. 1 daily (30)'.

A minute later he came in out of the garden carrying two cartons with six eggs in each.

'I'd like you to try my eggs,' he said shyly.

'That's very kind of you.' I took them. They were still warm and a small brown feather was stuck to one. He helped me get the cabinet into the back seat of the VW.

'I'll look in in a week and tell you how the speaker's

working and see how you are. Thanks for the eggs. Now, you will get the prescription made up straight away won't you? Let me have the card filled in when I see you, OK?'

I guessed it would be no good telling him to come to the surgery, which would have been normal routine. I dropped the cabinet at the surgery to keep it as a surprise and, incidentally, to give it a coat of varnish before revealing it to Elisabeth.

We had an egg each all round for tea – they were good! Deep orange yolks and whites like curdled milk, they were so fresh.

'Why don't you get Mr Butterworth to supply us regularly?' said Elisabeth.

'I'll see if he can when I go next week to see about his treatment.'

I hadn't let on about the primary purpose of my visiting him but she was within an ace of finding out next morning when she told our home help, Mrs Clout, about the eggs.

'Buttercup Joe!' exploded that good lady. 'He's a proper card, he is. Does people's wirelesses as well as keeping hens. Never sends them bills and often lends them sets while theirs is mending – which can be for the duration! I even heard of someone selling Joe back his own set because theirs never got mended.'

When she told me, I hoped inwardly that my speaker wasn't someone else's. Or at any rate, if it had been, that it was so far in the past as to be forgotten.

It was just three days before Christmas when I dropped in on Buttercup Joe again. It was amazing – and gratifying. Even in a week his voice was clearer and more normal in pitch, his skin a little less baggy and his pulse was sixty-five. He still wore his overcoat at all times however.

'How d'you feel, Mr Butterworth?'

His eyes positively twinkled.

'Better, thank you,' and then, 'I must say, there's something to be said for you doctors after all.'

He had a dozen eggs ready and tried to make me take them as a present again, but I refused and paid him his price

– about a shilling a dozen less than the shop price for the mass-produced article.

The back door banged and a female voice called, 'Joe, where are you?' Then a sturdy woman with healthy red cheeks and bright brown eyes walked in.

'Oh I'm sorry,' she said, stepping back into the doorway.

'Don't mind me,' I said, 'I'm Doctor Hamilton – just going.'

Buttercup Joe was giving a very good impression of a callow youth caught kissing in the hen-house.

'May I introduce Miss Lucy Elphinstone, my fiancée?'

'Very pleased to meet you, Miss Elphinstone,' I said.

'And you too, doctor,' she replied with surprising warmth.

'Well, I must be off. See you after Christmas, Mr Butterworth.'

Buttercup Joe went out to his kitchen, but Miss Elphinstone came with me to the door.

'Whatever have you given him, doctor?' she whispered. 'We've been courting for five years and he didn't pop the question till yesterday!'

'I think perhaps his condition has made him slow up in many ways – including getting down to the question of marriage!' I answered. 'Goodbye now.'

I strode down the path.

I was just getting into the car when she came running after me.

'Doctor, hope you won't mind me asking, but do you attend Mrs Charles of Beresford Farm?'

'Yes, I do as a matter of fact. Why?'

'She's just been brought into hospital by ambulance. I work there as a sort of land-girl and she collapsed in the yard this morning, so I rang for an ambulance and they took her in. Her husband was away for the day at a sale, but I got a message to him. I expect he's at the hospital by now – I thought perhaps you wouldn't have heard yet.'

'Thank you for letting me know. I'll go and see her.'

I closed the car door. I remembered Freda Charles. She was a tall, quiet, madonna-like lady – an unexpected sort of wife for Eddie Charles. He was a rough, bruiser-like specimen, but not lacking in a kind of swashbuckling attractiveness.

I found she'd already had the operation when I got to the Duke of Gloucester.

'Ruptured ovarian cyst,' said the sister laconically. 'Fortunately, not too much bleeding, should do OK. She's still very dopey.'

I decided to come back later. However, it was Christmas Eve before I managed it.

Mrs Charles was lying quietly propped up on her pillows, her pallor deeper than ever. Blood from the bottle hanging on a stand dripped steadily into a vein in her arm. There was something about her – a look of resignation – a languor which I couldn't attribute solely to the shock of her operation.

I smiled at her and sat quietly by her bed for a few moments before speaking.

'Feeling pretty low?'

She nodded and then, to my surprise, tears welled up in her large, dark eyes and rolled down her cheeks.

It took me completely aback – she was always so composed and in control of her emotions. Awkwardly, I reached out, grabbed a packet of tissues and handed her two of them. She dabbed her eyes and tried to smile. Then she spoke quietly, her voice straining from the effect of the tracheal tube through which she had been breathing the anaesthetic. Her words shook me.

'Doctor, my husband is leaving me.'

In short sentences she told me the pitiful story: her husband's rumbustiousness, his growing irritation with her quietness and composure; her attempts to meet his sexual demands, then her frequent attacks of abdominal pain and disinclination for sex relations; the predictable sequel – a barn dance at a local farm, the vivacious, flighty daughter of the house whom he fell for and was now openly associating with, and his announcement just before her attack that he was leaving. He had paid a cursory visit to the hospital yesterday but appeared unbending in his decision.

'Never accept one side of a family quarrel before you hear the other.' Charles's words drummed in my ears, but I couldn't help a burning indignation with this chap from welling up inside me as I looked at his wife, who could easily have died on the operating-table the day before. The resources of strength she needed for recovery were now being undermined by this impending catastrophe in her life.

It was Christmas Eve; Elisabeth would be dressing our little Christmas tree once the kids were in bed, but I had to do something about this situation – and do it now.

I got Miss Spencer to ring home for me to say I'd be a bit late after surgery and, thank goodness, it was for once a light session. I loaded the cabinet speaker into the back seat and drove out over the Downs to Beresford Farm. It was taking a chance – he might be off somewhere, but I didn't fancy giving him warning. As I turned in through the white gate-posts, I saw there was a light in the barn. I pulled up in front of it and Eddie Charles came out to see who was arriving at that time of night.

'What are you doing here, doc? The wife isn't worse is she?'

There was genuine anxiety in his voice, and I took heart.

'No, Mr Charles, she's doing all right – the operation's been quite successful so far, but I would like a word with you if you can give me the time.'

He looked at me curiously.

'Rather. Come into the house, doc. Have a glass of sherry?' he asked, as we went into the timbered sitting-room.

'No thanks, I've got a high tea waiting for me at home.'

There was nothing for it. I said straight out that his wife had broken down and told me that he was going to leave her. I wanted to do something to help, but only if he wished it. He would need to tell me his side of the story first, however. He must try to look on me as a friend as well as a doctor and take me into his confidence.

I'll say this, he didn't excuse himself. He'd found himself getting irritated by his wife's composure for a long time – he called it her superiority and aloofness. (Maybe there was a bit of hidden resentment here – she did come from a rather different social background.) 'I'm just a simple working farmer, doc,' he said.

Perhaps he'd been a bit demanding sexually, but she'd never refused him until recently and of course she'd had the pain – but then he'd thought at first it was a bit of a put-on.

I listened, not saying anything in condemnation. At last he ran out of words and he sat, hands on the knees of his riding breeches, looking into the fire.

I put up a silent prayer for help. After all, I thought, I'm not a marriage guidance counsellor. I knew in my heart that what cemented Elisabeth's and my relationship wasn't only affinity of mind or sexual love, it was a common focal point in Jesus Christ. But where was I to start with Eddie Charles? 'Better begin with your failures – not your successes, old chap,' I told myself.

So I tried first to identify with him in his temptation to be interested in other women. I had to fight it too – I failed often in my thoughts and I had to put things right with Elisabeth. We were on common ground here. I talked of the binding of a marriage being more than just sex – important though that was. Then I spoke of the children: they'd a boy at prep school and a girl away at boarding school, and they were desperately dependent on a stable home. I told him what his wife had finally said to me – that she loved him dearly but sometimes her reserve prevented her from showing it, and I didn't stop short of pulling the heart-strings a bit, picturing her fighting to recover and needing his help.

It was getting late. I stood up.

'Thank you for coming anyway, doc – on Christmas Eve too.' He lit the path to the car with a torch and stood for a few moments with head bowed in the headlights as I moved away.

As I drove along the lane I felt suddenly tired and sick. What a mess I'd made of it. Preaching at the man – maybe I'd put the tin lid on the whole affair. I'd broken *every* rule of marriage guidance – well, the few I knew. I'd gone to his home uninvited, I'd used moral persuasion, I'd – goodness, what hadn't I done? What a way to spend Christmas Eve.

Elisabeth was a bit glum when I got in but when I explained, she put her arms round my neck and kissed me (which she doesn't often do) and I felt better.

I helped her finish the children's stockings and put the final decorations on the tree, and we went to bed. On Christmas morning, I managed to sneak out to the car while Elisabeth was in the bathroom, and put the cabinet in the lounge. I wonder how many wives would have shown such appreciation on being given a bit of old junk for Christmas, but she did, and when we connected it up, the Christmas music really came over beautifully.

It was a happy day – not too spoilt by my having to go out to see a young man. His wife's message was that 'he'd-come-home-in-a-collapsed-state-and-she-couldn't-get-him-off-the-floor-and-could-I-come-at-once'. I admit that it's difficult to lift a hefty young fellow up when he's dead drunk, but between us we dumped him on the bed to sleep it off. It meant that we all missed the Christmas morning service. We heard the Queen's speech on the new speaker after Christmas dinner, played charades and party games and showed the children a Christmas film-strip before they went to bed. Then we sat on our own by the fire thinking of other Christmases in Africa and England.

Three weeks later I had a card from Torquay which simply said 'Thanks' and was signed 'Eddie and Freda Charles'.

Each time I saw Buttercup Joe he had improved. He only wore an overcoat outside now. His face became thinner and healthier, his eyes twinkled with a roguish glint. He tried every way to get me to take his eggs without paying, but when he failed, he resorted to picking out all of the double yolks which were so gigantic they must have made the birds that laid them say 'ouch' each time.

In the early spring, he and Lucy were married at a Register Office.

I wondered how she would cope with his radio museum but, after all, she did know what she was letting herself in for. Buttercup Joe was just an incurable magpie. He collected and then couldn't let things go – of course, at times people like me were grateful to find something useful in the chaos.

To my surprise, it seemed that order was gradually being created at Buttercup Joe's, and the volume of old cabinets was shrinking by imperceptible degrees. One day Lucy let me in on the secret.

'When he's out on his egg-round, I burn one old set a day in the garden. He doesn't seem to notice!'

I guessed otherwise. A love like his that had taken so long to mature was impervious to such minor attacks as the loss of some of his magpie hoard.

Happily it became apparent very soon that a new little Buttercup would soon be blooming. With Joe over fifty and Lucy a mere ten years younger, they must have felt there was no time to lose.

Her pregnancy was surprisingly uneventful. Lucy and Joe were adamant that the baby must be born at home. As an elderly primip, Lucy should have gone to hospital for the birth. It was a long drawn-out process which ended in a forceps delivery, but Joe number two appeared unharmed apart from a bruised ear. The midwife and I won the battle – but I lost another.

From that day to this, I have never been able to pay Buttercup Joe for a single egg.

20

Boats

'Crazy! No other word for it! Calls 'imself a doctor? It's 'is 'ead needs examinin'. Fancy taking 'is missus an' 'is kid on a day like that, an' no other boats out nor nothin'. Crazy. That's what it was.'

It was coming over loud and clear as I crossed the garage to where my car was standing, perched on a ramp in the corner.

The voice went on: 'Can't take no liberties with the sea, got to know what you're doin', you 'ave. Don't suppose 'e'd ever been sailing before. I tell you, I've been fishin' for years an' it scares the pants off me often. Hey! What you kickin' me for? Oh! Sorry sir, didn't see you was there. Car's nearly ready, won't keep you more 'an a minute or two.'

The head mechanic ducked out from under the Volkswagen where he'd been adjusting the brakes and glowered red-faced at his assistant who'd been trying to stem the flow of comment, seeing my approach.

He squinted cautiously at me from under the peak of his oily army surplus cap.

'Never mind, Alf,' I said. 'No offence, you're bang on – it was crazy. I should never have gone out like that without taking proper precautions.'

It all started with that paragraph in the small ads section of the local paper: '*National 12. Half-built. Prepared timber sufficient to complete. £30 o.n.o. Brown, 15 Sea View Road, evenings only.*'

From the moment we arrived in Wilverton it had been our ambition to have a boat. It was such a waste – all that sea and nothing to sail on it. For sailing was in the blood. I think I can claim precedence since I have a photograph of my father sailing on the Clyde with me sitting in the bottom of the boat still in nappies. My grandfather was chief engineer on the steam yacht of the Khedive of Egypt, but perhaps that doesn't count.

Elisabeth has sailed boats ever since she was a teenager, and owned a fourteen-foot dinghy on the Cam. Her boating lineage goes farther than mine, as an ancestor of hers was boatswain on the *Royal Yacht Catherine* around 1650.

It could be said that sailing was what spliced us because soon after I'd met Elisabeth I asked if I could sail her boat *The Vixen* with her. Unwisely she agreed. We were on the Cam half-way up Ditton reach, with me at the helm, when I tried a turn with the sheet too tight and capsized us. We had no buoyancy in those days. Standing up to her chest in mud and water, with weed in her hair, her only comment was, 'Better get the sail down'. I felt at that moment, 'This is the girl for me!'

A National 12 was not quite what we'd visualized – a bit too racy and unstable for a family. But beggars can't be choosers. Even a second-hand boat could have been around £100, and I only had £20 to spare.

'It does say "or near offer" Elisabeth – do you think £20 is near enough?'

'I should have a try,' she advised.

I went round that evening.

A cheery young fellow about my own age took me down to the basement.

'To tell you the truth I started building her before the war. Then I got called up, and had to abandon the job. Never got going again after the war, got married and moved off down the coast. She's been in here ever since. Perfectly dry, mind you. All I can say is the wood must be well seasoned by now. Dad's retired and wants the basement for garden tools, now he's concentrating on the great outdoors.' He threw open the door. 'There she lies!'

The boat was still a mere shell completed up to the gunwales and standing on wooden formers. By the wall lay a stack of various sizes of timber, dusty but tidily arranged. He picked up a roughly shaped rudder and stroked it lovingly.

'Look at that! Specially selected mahogany – grain goes with the curve – it'll never snap. Not the collapsible sort though, I'm afraid – wasn't thought of in 1938!'

'How do we get it out then?' I asked.

The passage between the houses was very narrow.

He laughed. 'No problem. Neighbour's given me permission to take down a section of her fence.'

I felt I must now make my position clear.

'I'd like to buy the boat, but I can only go to £20.'

He looked at me for a moment. 'OK, it's a deal. I'll be honest. I haven't had another offer. People don't want the sweat of building. A kit's all right, just shove it together, but real carpentry – nothing doing. And this design – authentic Uffa Fox mind you – is a bit out of date. But she'll sail, I promise you. Well, best of luck.'

'I'll let you know when I can collect,' I told him, as we parted in the road.

I drove home, my head full of delightful romantic visions.

We could teach the children to sail for a start; maybe we might even sail along the coast and picnic in some isolated cove or take it on the river for camping holidays. The unstable twelve-footer grew in my imagination into a small cabin cruiser. It was a boat, a real boat, and it was ours – well nearly. The last one I'd owned had been in Kenya, a canoe which I had planned to use for a safari up the Kerio River to Lake Rudolph. That was an unfulfilled dream.

I hadn't been home long that evening before it began to look as if this was another one. Elisabeth listened to my description. Her eyes looked doubtful. I could see she was having second thoughts.

'How are you going to finish it, Andy dear? You don't get all that much free time, and you know your best carpentry's been done with a hatchet!'

I felt distinctly deflated.

'Oh, come off it! It's not as bad as all that!'

But I knew it was. Give me an axe and I could build a hut with poles cut from the African forest with anyone. But this was indeed a job for a real *fundi*, which is an expressive Swahili word for an expert.

Next morning when I told Charles about the boat, I could see there was more than a flicker of interest but he didn't offer any comment at first. He kindly turned down the rumpled collar of my jacket in his annoying way and then, in a typical offhand manner, he said, 'I wouldn't mind having a bash at it myself – provided you help, of course.'

'Charles, would you really? That's a very sporting offer.'

Carpentry came as easily to Charles as the classics. My spirits rose.

'You know that shed behind the garage?' he went on. 'We could park it there for a month or two.'

'I'm just wondering how I can get her up to your house.'

'Well, I leave that up to you Andy. But when you fix it, let me know.'

If I'd known anyone with a trailer, I could have borrowed it for the occasion – provided they lent me their car as well – but I didn't.

Then help came from an unexpected quarter. There was

a young plumber called Nigel doing some jobs in the surgery. He was tightening up the outlet pipe from the basin in my room and I was telling him about the boat, as I knew he had a small fishing boat of his own.

'I could give you a hand, doc. Besides, I know a bloke in the removal business. I'll get him to pick up your dinghy on a return trip. Wouldn't cost you much.'

'Nigel – you're my fairy godmother!'

He grinned at the unlikely epithet as he gripped his pipe-wrench in a pair of brawny hands and bent to his task. 'Always ready to help a fellow seafarer,' he laughed.

Later we fixed an evening to coincide with the removal man and I let the boat-owner know.

We had to take a section of the fence down, as he had predicted. Even then it was a dreadful job getting the hull out of the basement door and up the passageway to the road. It was a lot heavier than it looked. We carted up all spare timber and stacked it on the footpath. Then we replaced the fencing and bolted it in place.

It was just five minutes to four. The van was promised for four o'clock. At half past four we were still waiting.

'Must have got hung up on the job,' grunted Nigel.

I was getting a bit anxious. 'Look Nigel, I'm afraid I've got a surgery at half past five. What d'you suggest? Should we take it all back?'

The idea was not exactly exhilarating.

'What? Put that fence down and up again? Hump that boat back? Not on your life!'

He sized me up. 'Look here doc, what about taking it ourselves? Not all that far is it?'

'OK, Nigel. I'm game if you are.'

We quickly stacked the spare wood and formers back in the basement and bent to the hull.

'Hup!' said Nigel, and we heaved it aloft together. It wasn't done as dextrously as the Boat Race oarsmen do it, but there are eight of them!

I was at the sharp end and the keel settled fairly comfortably into the hollow of my shoulder. All went well until we left Sea View and steered crabwise into the main street. As we trudged along in the gutter to avoid ramming passers-by, a bus overhauled us. As it came abreast the driver flipped open his window and shouted, 'Wot, no water? Haw Haw!'

I got such a start that I didn't notice the bus stop sign. I'm afraid a little repainting of the post will be needed about five feet up. Poor Nigel got a nasty jolt twelve feet astern. 'Watch it, doc!' he yelped.

My shoulder was aching by the time we reached the crossroads. The policeman on point duty was fortunately one of our patients. Very kindly he held up the traffic for us to cross. Even he couldn't resist a wisecrack: 'Why don't you try rowing it?'

We found we were steadily collecting a string of small boys on the pavement who kept pace beside us, keeping up a running commentary. I'd changed to my left shoulder and my head was on the far side of the boat from them. The leader ran forward, looked back and yelled at his mates.

'It's my doctor!'

He walked backwards grinning at me.

'It ain't the carnival for six weeks, doc, you've got the wrong date!'

'Buzz off, Kevin, will you? I'll give you some really nasty medicine the next time you're in the surgery, so watch it!'

He laughed raucously, but he was a decent lad and he hauled off the gang, and they dropped astern.

I was just beginning to wish I'd never seen that wretched advert when Charles's gateway hove in sight. Wearily we 'put our helm down', did a neat tack into the drive and almost trotted into the open shed to lower the boat thankfully to the floor.

Nigel rubbed his shoulder.

'Not to worry about the wood, doc. I'll pick it up in my little van.'

I stopped swinging my arm round to ease the pain in the supraspinatus muscle.

'Thanks a lot Nigel, I'm very grateful. You've been a tremendous help.'

'Any time, doc.'

Charles really enjoyed himself completing the construction

of that boat. He did a beautiful job. I held planks in place, and was even allowed to put in an occasional brass screw or copper nail. He fashioned mast, gaff and boom out of the pine; gunwales and rubbing strakes out of larch, ribs of steamed oak. Thwarts and the knee brackets, whose nautical name I can't remember, were made out of mahogany.

I answered an advert for second-hand sails. Charles felt that ease of transport and stability would be enhanced, even if we lost a bit of speed, if we rigged it as a Heron, to reduce the sail area and the height of the mast. This enabled us to use marine ply for the centre-board instead of a heavy steel. Ships' chandlers near the harbour supplied manilla rope, cleats and wire for the shrouds. I helped to put on the three coats of marine varnish over the hull, rudder and spars.

After two months of hard spare-time work, Charles announced that she was ready for launching.

By this time I'd found a sailing club friend with a trailer. He kindly used his Ford to tow us down to the harbour. Elisabeth, surprisingly, volunteered to come with me. I think she didn't trust me on my own. At the last minute Sarah, who had the afternoon off school, begged to be allowed to come too. Very reluctantly we agreed. We had a selection of old kapok-filled lifebelts, and a whole series of rubber tubes and floats to act as buoyancy bags.

Now, I have no excuse for the chapter of errors and omissions that heralded our first little voyage. I can only explain it by saying that I was in a state of mild euphoria at the prospect of actually getting the boat on the water. We slid the dinghy off the trailer on to the harbour slipway and dragged it into the water.

An old fisherman standing in the lee of the jetty took his pipe out and surveyed us.

'Better keep a weather eye open when ye gits outside.'

'Thank you.'

I was beginning to feel a little nervous, and this wasn't helped by our finding our feet awash as soon as we pushed off. I hadn't screwed in the stoppers for the bilge drainage-holes. I leant over the stern and corrected this omission.

Elisabeth took the tiller and mainsheet. I hauled the jib tight and Sarah sat on the floor near the mast and we were off.

We got the meaning of the fisherman's message when we cleared the harbour-arm. Although it was a lovely sunny May day, there was a fair breeze from the east and a popple on the water. We were cramped in the boat designed for two, so we'd left the oars behind and simply took a paddle.

With a following wind we ran down the front for about a mile at about five hundred yards off the shore. It was very pleasant, the little craft responded well to the rudder, it didn't seem over-canvassed and rode the waves without shipping water. I was lulled into an unwarranted feeling of security.

'Time to turn – remember we've got to tack back.'

Elisabeth's words broke in on my thoughts.

'Lee-ho!'

She turned her expertly and we started to beat out to sea.

'Can I take over the tiller, darling?'

We exchanged places and when I'd got my leg disentangled from the mainsheet we were on our way quite smoothly again.

Then – it was almost a re-run of our first sail on the Cam. The wind freshened, we were in the trough of a wave and as we swept up to the crest there was a sudden gust. I had the mainsail too close-hauled and in a second we were over. Sarah screamed but she was all right. Cold though the water was, our lifebelts held us up.

Elisabeth held on to her while I stood on the centre-board and slowly the dinghy righted itself. But the buoyancy was far too little and she floated submerged to the gunwales. Elisabeth and Sarah clambered in. The wet sail swayed the boat wildly in the breeze and she nearly went over again, so Elisabeth unhitched the mainsail halyard and dropped the sail. I hung on to the bow – to have climbed in would have sunk them.

'Where's the bailer?'

Where indeed? One more error! It had not been tied on and presumably it was now on the bottom. The paddle too was gone, it must have floated away in the confusion. So

162

there we were – waterlogged, sails down and no way of bailing or getting towards the shore as we couldn't hoist the sail in case of another capsize.

As far as I could see, there were very few people about. We were far down the front and no one seemed to be taking any notice of our plight.

'Someone'll come out in a rowing boat or something, love,' I called to Elisabeth – but someone didn't. She and Sarah must have been cold, soaked to the skin and in the breeze, but in the water I was getting pretty frigid. In early May the sea around Britain hasn't got much heat in it. Gradually my legs got heavy and I kicked to keep them alive and also to drive our little craft nearer the shore.

Suddenly we heard it in the distance. 'Bang' and then again 'Bang'. It was the lifeboat call. As we learnt afterwards, one pair of eyes – a very elderly pair – had been watching us and they were wise old eyes too.

Our old patient Miss Celia Beckwith, for whom Algernon had done a night duty and whose sister had now passed on, had more time on her hands. She had been studying the Channel shipping through a pair of old binoculars. Suddenly our little dinghy had sailed into view and she saw the whole episode. She hadn't a telephone but, infirm as she was, she had struggled downstairs from her flat on the front and along to a telephone box, dialled 999 and alerted the lifeboat station.

Having heard the bangs, we waited for our rescue with mixed feelings of relief and apprehension for causing all this trouble. At last, round the harbour-arm came the lifeboat. Its bow-wave built up and in no time she was lying to, to windward of us, engine throbbing. A boat-hook hauled us alongside and we were aboard. It was warm down below. They gave us blankets and even a mug of hot soup each. Before we'd finished it, we were back in harbour.

The coxswain was very nice and said little in response to my apologies for getting them out.

'We have to look after all sorts, sir,' was his somewhat cryptic reply.

Our dinghy had been partly bailed out and towed in. The

crew beached her and my pal picked her up that evening and brought her up to 'Salud'. We were taken home in a taxi.

On the way, I began to feel rather odd. I felt my pulse – it was fast and irregular. I realized that the chilling and exertion in the water had given my ticker a bit of a beating.

It took two days to settle down by which time I had gained a lot more sympathy for the worries of fit people suddenly taken ill. It was very humbling having to accept that I wasn't physically invincible – something dear Elisabeth had learnt about herself long before.

To complete the process of putting me in my place, *The Wilverton Advertiser* accorded me a headline: 'Local doctor involved in sea drama with wife and daughter', and continued: 'Tells our reporter "I should have known better".'

That just about sums it up.

21
'After the sun the rain'

I sat there, sucking the top of my biro, gazing into space. The day had started badly. My *amour propre* had suffered a body blow . . .

She had come late, without an appointment. Her appearance suggested what my mother used to describe as 'having been pulled through a hedge backwards'. Untidy hair, make-up slapped on at random, nail varnish peeling off, cardigan buttoned in the wrong holes, nylons wrinkled.

But her face was vaguely familiar. Yes, she was the lady in the sweet shop on the front, who had served me with a gallon of ice-cream for our boys' club New Year party. Now she had a five-year-old son with her.

'Doctor, he's not eating proper, just doesn't want his food.'

For a half-starved child, he looked remarkably well nourished. He wasn't lacking in energy either and he proceeded to use some of it up on the surgery equipment, blandly disregarded by his mum. Just in time I seized him before he could truncate the curtains with a pair of my surgical scissors.

Drawing on all my reserves of patience and persuasion, I managed to get him to submit to a cursory examination. When he opened his mouth he revealed a half-sucked sweet on his tongue, staining it a repulsive green. His primary dentition was badly decayed. As I let him go, he popped another sweet into his mouth from the bag in his hand.

I looked sternly at his mother.

'Mrs Webster, I should say Ian's trouble is simply too many sweets. They've caused tooth decay and they're no doubt taking away his appetite for proper food. That's all that's wrong with him, Mrs Webster. Cut out his sweets.'

I wasn't prepared for her instant verbal retaliation.

'It's very fine for you doctors, sitting there all splendid, acting high and mighty and telling us what to do. You should try having a few kids of your own to look after single-handed. You'd give 'em sweets to keep 'em quiet!'

She grabbed her offspring's hand and stormed out of the surgery, leaving the door wide open.

'Do I really give that impression?' I wondered.

True – more than once Charles has suggested that I display an overweening confidence in my own rectitude. And that word 'splendid' struck a particularly unpleasant chord of memory. In a flash of enlightenment I now thought I understood why my rugger team-mates at Cambridge had called me 'Splendid Andy'. Splendid Andy – had I changed so little in twenty years? Was I still so splendid in my own eyes? I was downcast.

Mrs Webster's outburst hadn't been the first upset of the day, for it was scheduled as Barney's first one at school.

Sarah's scholastic establishment boasted a kindergarten and thither we proceeded after breakfast. Barney had been hankering after going to school like his big sister and brother for a long time but, when it came to the point, he just wouldn't get out of the car.

'Don't wanna go to school today, Daddy. Wanna go home,' he wailed.

'Now Barney, you've got to go. They're waiting for you; they're ever so kind – you'll like it. Sarah does.'

But it was no good. We drove round once to give him time and then came back, but he was adamant. 'Not goin' to school,' he announced and his face had that obstinate look. He must get it from Elisabeth.

There was nothing for it. I had to carry him in, feeling like a callous brute. I shuddered as I thought of the look of reproach on Barney's tear-stained countenance as I turned away and left him.

Little did that Mrs Webster know of her medical adviser's own family crises . . .

It was a positive relief when the telephone broke in on my unpleasant reverie.

'There's a Doctor Farjeon who would like to speak to you. Will you take the call?' It was Miss Spencer.

Farjeon? Surely not Neil Farjeon – it was back during the war when we'd last met. 'Put him through please. Doctor Andrew Hamilton here.'

'Hullo, Andy – it's been a long time!' I recognized the same slow, whimsical voice.

'Neil! What are you doing in Wilverton? I thought you were in South India.'

'We're on leave and we arranged a holiday with the family. We're staying at "The Limes". Do you know it?'

'Of course, I must come round.'

'Well, Andy, if you do, I wonder if you could have a look at Eileen. She's not been herself lately; it would be kind, if you can manage it.'

'I'll be with you after surgery – say half an hour. OK?'

It sounds pretentious but I think many doctors develop a special sensitivity to the *cri de coeur* – however faint it may be. Whether I'm right or not, something in Neil's unemotional words convinced me that Eileen and he were in great need of help.

I looked forward to seeing them again, though the thought of our last meeting did nothing to re-establish my self-esteem.

On that occasion they hadn't long come home on leave. It was in the middle of the war and they couldn't get back to

India. Neil was filling in in a practice in Worcestershire where the doctor had joined the services, and when my friend John and I arrived in the locality to do a paediatric course in an evacuated hospital, we found our promised billet already filled.

Neil and Eileen immediately offered us the use of their spare bedroom.

I wasn't as quick in medical uptake as John, and while he snored in the bed next to mine, I mugged up my textbook on children in the night hours. To avoid disturbing him one night, I hung a rugger sock over the bedside light to shade it from his eyes.

I woke shivering at 2 a.m. and became aware of a haze in the bedroom and an appalling smell. A charred sock hung in remnants on the light and a long black streak of soot stained the distempered wall almost to the ceiling. Only redecoration would ever hide it.

Eileen was very sweet about it. John showed rather less understanding – after all, it was his sock.

I drove into the drive of 'The Limes'. The proprietress showed me up to their room. Neil opened the door. He had aged, but the crow's-feet at the corners of his eyes only accentuated their steady kindness.

'Great to see you Andy – what is it – twelve or thirteen years?'

'I can't tell you what it means to me to link up, Neil,' I answered. 'You were so good to us during the war. I'm sorry Eileen's unwell. Fancy you landing up with me of all people, for a second opinion! Any idea of the trouble?'

He frowned and compressed his lips.

'It's difficult to say,' he said slowly. 'You know how it is when you live together – you don't notice gradual changes, especially if you're doctors! No, there's nothing much to go on – she's simply had no energy for several weeks. Of course the journey's been tiring, but now for the first time she says she's got pain, low down in the tummy and it doesn't go. I'll be grateful if you'll have a look. She's expecting you and she's so pleased you could make it. Now don't worry about the children – they're big enough to look after themselves and they're down on the beach. They won't disturb us. Come and see her.'

He opened the door of the next room and led the way.

Eileen was sitting up in bed with a welcoming smile.

'Hullo, Andy! Same old tough guy! Still playing rugger?'

I shook my head.

'I'm hoping Peter will carry on where I left off – I'm too old for the game now. But what's all this? I'm sorry to hear you're not well. What have you got to tell me?'

I was trying to show a joviality I did not feel. Neil went out silently and closed the door.

I sat down on the edge of the bed. Eileen too was going grey I noted. She had always worn spectacles; behind them, her grey eyes looked hollow and tired. Her cheeks had lost the colour I remembered they had always had in the past. I felt in my bones that something was seriously wrong.

She told me briefly of an inexplicable weariness which had increased for some weeks and then this nagging low abdominal pain had started. That was all.

General examination was negative. Then I did an internal. In the left fornix of the vagina there was a mass, and it was binding the pelvic structures together.

I washed my hands at the basin and as I turned, drying them on a towel, I saw she was watching me.

'Well, Andy – what's the verdict?' Eileen was a doctor and a brave, well-balanced person. There would be no stalling.

'There's a resistance in the left fornix. I feel you must see a gynaecologist. I really can't go further than that at present.

For a moment her eyes clouded and I saw her lower lip tremble. She held it in her teeth.

'Neil dear,' she called. He came in and crossed the room to take the hand she held out to him. 'Would you tell Neil what you found, please, Andy?'

He sat still, on the edge of the bed, just looking at Eileen as I repeated my findings. The feeling of their oneness was almost palpable.

A business-like approach was the thing now, I decided.

'Of course, we don't know what we've got to deal with as

yet. Would you like to see a local consultant or go up to your old hospital?' Eileen had trained at the Royal Free.

She replied at once. 'Oh, could I see your local man? It would spoil the children's holiday if we had to leave now and go off to London. Let's see what he says and then, if I need to, I could go up to the Royal Free afterwards.'

Jefferson, the local gynaecologist, was very co-operative. He came round that afternoon. My suspicions were confirmed.

'Almost certainly, carcinoma of the left ovary with local spread. Must have a laparotomy as soon as possible.'

We contacted the Royal Free. The Farjeons managed one day with both our families at our beach-hut, finished their week's holiday, and off they went. I had a preliminary report after her operation. It was an inoperable cancer, she was very poorly post-operatively and stayed in hospital. Weeks went by and I heard nothing. Then, two months later, I was notified of her death and a full report was enclosed.

Eileen had deteriorated rapidly. Then, six weeks after the operation, there had been a massive internal haemorrhage from an eroded blood vessel and she had died suddenly.

Neil's letter followed, giving his personal account of her stay in hospital.

'. . . When the initial shock wore off, Eileen showed an amazing spirit. She hardly talked about herself at all . . . she planned the future for the children and me. She even insisted that if I could find the right one, I should get married again for my own sake and the children's . . . I can only praise God for her.'

It was restrained and courageous, but his heart-break and lostness were there to be read between the lines. He thanked me for my help. He felt he should stay in England and try to build a home-life for the children.

As I put down the single sheet of notepaper, a line I learnt in childhood came into my head quite unbidden: 'After the sun the rain.'

I have an unsophisticated taste in literature and in spite of having to read Dickens under duress at school, I thoroughly enjoy his novels still. I savour the sonorous dialogue and the stylized scenes, and even snigger at the bold contrivance of his characters and plots. But something happened to me in real life that was pure Dickens.

It was roughly a year after the Farjeons' sad little holiday in Wilverton, that I had another visit from Mrs Webster, the lady with the unruly child. Even before she sat herself down I could see there was something different in her manner.

She hadn't lost her faculty for speaking her mind however.

'Doctor, I want to say I'm sorry for blowing my top when I came with Ian.'

'That's OK, Mrs Webster. I expect I was a bit aggressive in the way I spoke to you.'

'Would you have a look at my hands, doctor?' I found she had a nasty weeping eczema of the fingers, chiefly involving the left hand.

'Do you use a lot of detergents in the washing-up?'

'Yes, doctor.'

'Well, I'm afraid they're causing you trouble. I expect you put your left hand in the water more than the right, don't you?'

She did.

I advised wearing rubber gloves and gave her some hydro-cortisone cream to take away the inflammation of the skin. She took the prescription, but she didn't go.

'Could you spare me a moment doctor, there's something I want to tell you?'

She looked so earnest about it that I ignored the pile of record-cards on the desk and said, 'Please, carry on.'

She began: 'I was up in London seeing my mum, it was soon after I brought Ian to see you.' She gave me a wry little smile. 'I got taken with this terrible pain in my stomach. I knew I'd fallen for another baby, but I didn't expect anything like this just from being pregnant. I never had trouble like it when I was carrying Ian. Anyway, Mum got her doctor and he sent me straight into the Royal Free Hospital. I was real bad. The gynaecologist specialist said I'd got an egg-topic. Sounds like a new ice-cream, don't it? Anyway I was past caring. They doped me and took me to the operating theatre. Afterwards, he explained that the baby had lodged outside the womb and had sort of burst out internally. I'd lost a lot of blood and had to have a transfusion after the operation.

'Sorry to go on doctor – but I'm getting to it. Well, on the ward was this lady. Although she was a patient she was a doctor too, see? You could see she was really bad. This was the thing though. Even though she was so ill, she used to go round all the other patients cheering them up and when she couldn't get out of bed, they'd come to her just to have a talk, if they could make it.

'Now if ever there was a real Christian, she was. She didn't seem to have any fear though she must have known she wasn't going to get better, being a doctor, an' all. I began to wish I had a faith like hers. One day she gave me a little book about becoming a Christian.

'Doctor, that book really changed my life, that and seeing her. I feel I know Jesus for myself. Coo! It hasn't half changed things for Bert and me – even Ian seems a different boy. Sorry for taking up all your time doctor, but I felt I wanted to tell you – you being a missionary once and all that. I thought you'd be interested.'

'Mrs Farjeon, wasn't it?' I asked.

'Doctor! How did you know?'

'She and her husband were friends of mine, Mrs Webster. Thank you for telling me but I'm sure if she were here, she'd want to do something more to help you. Will you let me do it for her?'

I opened a drawer in the desk and took out a little booklet. It was a series of Bible readings with a straightforward commentary – one reading for each day. 'I use this sort of thing myself Mrs Webster. I find I've got to read a bit of the Bible every day to keep up my strength, just as I eat to keep the body going.'

I handed it to her. 'Would you like to have a look at it?'

She went out, and this time she shut the door quietly behind her.

The spring had come when we got a printed card in the post announcing the forthcoming marriage between Dr Neil Farjeon and Mrs Mary Wharton. Neil and Dick Wharton had been friends in the past. Dick was an army chaplain and went in with the troops on the Normandy landings. He was killed two days after D-Day. Mary had two children much of an age with Neil's. It had been a lonely life for her since the war.

Neil's brief letter with the card told us how he'd managed to rejoin the practice in Worcestershire as their senior partner was retiring and he would be setting up home there for them all, after the wedding.

'Come and burn a sock with us sometime,' he ended.

It gave me pleasure to contemplate two people turning tragedy into a new enterprise in love and understanding, where their children could mature in security.

I felt like finishing that verse which came to me on hearing of Eileen's death.

> After the sun the rain,
> After the rain the sun;
> This is the way of life,
> Till the work is done.

As I told Elisabeth, 'In a way, that just about sums it up for us too, love.'

'Yes, darling,' she said. Then her eyes twinkled. ' 'Fraid the work isn't done yet – I've a call for you . . .'

A Walk Across America
Peter Jenkins

This book is the story of the first half of Peter Jenkins' epic trek across America with his dog, Cooper. The author relives his moments of loneliness and exhilaration, and the varied experiences which changed his whole outlook—learning a mountain man's secret of survival, becoming part of an all-black community in North Carolina, working on a ranch in Alabama, sharing the lives of the many people he met:
'I had started out searching for myself and my country and found both. I came face to face with God and accepted him as my own.'

Journey to the Fourth World
Michael Cole

The Kali Gandaki is one of the world's most violent rivers. The people of Nepal call it 'the goddess of death'. But to the country's pioneering medical missionaries, it has always been seen as a potential highway through the mountains, linking homes with hospitals. Taking specially-designed new hovercraft, a 26-man British Joint Services Expedition set out to try to harness this previously unnavigable river. *Journey to the Fourth World* is the leader's account of this adventurous and testing expedition, and its results in and beyond Nepal.